SIMPSON THE OBSTETRICIAN

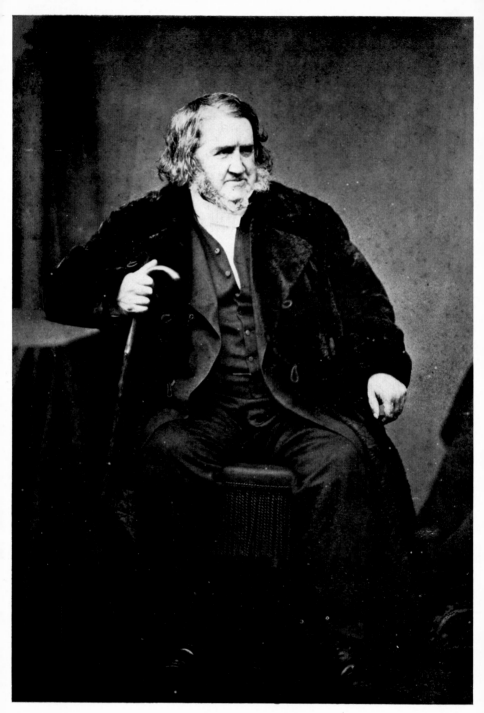

J. Y. Simpson as an old man

SIMPSON
THE OBSTETRICIAN

A biography

by

MYRTLE SIMPSON

LONDON
VICTOR GOLLANCZ
1972

ISBN 0 575 01368 0

Printed in Great Britain by
The Camelot Press Ltd., London and Southampton

One of the greatest legacies of any nation is the memory of a great man and the inheritance of a great example.

DISRAELI

Contents

List of Illustrations

Acknowledgements

I COULD NOT have put together this book without the memories of James Young Simpson's relations: Miss Katie Simpson, Mr Henry Drummond Simpson and my father-in-law, the Rev. Ian Grindlay Simpson. Their accumulation of newspaper cuttings, letters, and writings on the subject has been the source of much of my material.

Many eminent obstetricians have allowed me to make use of their writings, and, more important, their opinions; have readily given me of their time, answered questions and suggested books for me to read; these include Professor Ian Donald of Glasgow, Professor Chassar-Moir of Oxford, Dr J. A. Chalmers of Worcester and Dr Clifford Kennedy of Edinburgh. I am also grateful to the anaesthetist, Professor Cecil Gray, and to Mr John Shepherd, surgeon and historian, both of Liverpool.

I am extremely grateful to the Edinburgh Royal College of Physicians and particularly to their librarian, Miss Ferguson, who has filled great gaps in my knowledge. She has readily unearthed from the dust Simpson's own notebooks and manuscripts and I have enjoyed working in her magnificent library.

An enormous trunk of Simpson's own correspondence has been entrusted by his progeny to the care of the Edinburgh Royal College of Surgeons and I thank them for allowing me within their doors in order to read the family letters.

My mother-in-law, Dr Elenora Simpson, has helped me decipher reams of Victorian handwriting, and having been in the family longer than I, has assessed the Simpson image and compared it with that presented in my manuscript which she has also corrected.

In order to retain readability, references have not been interposed with the text. In a book such as this, verification has been necessary in nearly every instance, and the sources of my information are listed in the bibliography at the back of the book.

Concerning the illustrations, the National Portrait Gallery of Scotland has allowed me to use the photographs of young Simpson taken by Octavius Hill. I am very grateful for the privilege. Mrs Iitty Michaelson has assisted in their verification and given me advice.

This is a book about a man and the time in which he lived. It is not for me to assess his work; for that I am deeply grateful to Ian Donald, Regius Professor of Midwifery, University of Glasgow, who has written the Foreword.

M. S.

Foreword

HISTORY MAY BE remarkable for its ability to repeat itself, but is even more remarkable when it deals with something which can never be repeated. The mid period of the nineteenth century supplies such an instance.

Anaesthetic drugs, including laughing gas and ether, had already come earlier but the knowledge of their chemistry was not enough of itself. It required some dedicated fanatic like Simpson to force their use upon a profession none too ready then to change its methods and on a public whose philosophy still inclined it to think of pain as something purifying and not simply degrading as we now regard it.

What is most remarkable was that Simpson won through in the traditionally conservative field of midwifery rather than as a means of extending the scope of surgery which was a natural consequence. The idea that the pains of childbirth were God-given persisted into the days of my own father's rural general practice in Cornwall before the 1914–18 war.

Although Simpson had already tried ether in obstetrics, which is a safe though very disagreeable drug, he soon found in chloroform something that was both quick and not unpleasant. The fact that countless women died during the next hundred years, either directly or indirectly, from what is now regarded as an unacceptably dangerous anaesthetic does not lesson the importance of his great triumph.

There is much more to the story of Simpson, however. He wasted fewer minutes in his life than most men. He tilted at attitudes more formidable than windmills, and although what he did is exciting enough, the conditions and the prevailing philosophy of his time are more interesting still.

Had he lived in a different era he might have turned out differently but I think not. His mistakes, his quarrels, his reverence for the past, his fanaticism for the future, above all his vitality would not have been quenched in any other age. These features would all have shone through in his teaching whatever might have been his subject, since the art of teaching is the art of sharing enthusiasm.

Simpson was no scientist in the present sense, but a doctor, a doer and what the Scots call "a rare fechter".

His thinking got very near to the modern concept of asepsis which may account for his lack of excitement about the introduction of antisepsis, but in this he would have been ahead of Lister's contribution to surgery at that time.

To interest medical men, social historians and ordinary folk alike within the covers of one brief volume is an ambitious feat in scholarship and story telling. To maintain the sense of driving pressure throughout the account of this intense life is a literary challenge of some force. The reader can but judge the result, but through the pages there stands out the unique glory that was, and still is Edinburgh, capital city of Scotland.

Glasgow   IAN DONALD

Prologue

Edinburgh: Friday, 13 May 1870

EDINBURGH IN THE spring is crisp and clear. The hills that limit the horizon in every direction stand out sharp against the pale blue sky. 13 May 1870 was a chilly morning, with a northeast wind breathing across the Firth of Forth. The low northern sun had not much heat, but it gleamed on the stone buildings of the grey city with a soft light, and winked off the brass handles on the doors on the New Town streets. Splashes of colour also relieved the monochrome of the city: flags flying from the opulent shops of Princes Street, from the City Chambers, from the Castle itself.

However, the flags flew at half mast. It was the day of the funeral, and the city was gathering together as one man to demonstrate its feelings of private personal loss. Had it poured with rain, the people of Edinburgh would still have turned out in their thousands to pay their respects.

The University closed its classrooms at noon, students and staff scurried off in the same direction, down the Mound and into the New Town. The Stock Exchange suspended its transactions. As two o'clock drew near the general business of the city was brought to a halt and a feeling of impressive stillness settled over the usually active streets. The deep bell of St Giles began to toll, the notes picked up by lesser churches all over the town, quickening the feeling of a national loss.

Outside No. 52 Queen Street members of the public had begun to gather fully an hour before the procession was due to start. By two o'clock these had merged into one vast crowd, completely filling the wide, cobbled street and overflowing downhill along the intended route of the procession.

Meanwhile groups had also been collecting in other parts of the town. The University Court and Senate assembled in their robes and caps and filed up behind the bearers of the Mace, which had been covered in black crêpe. Behind them were lined up eighty Fellows of the Royal College, the sky-blue of the Physicians mingling with the dark-blue of the Surgeons. The entire Town Council had assembled in St Luke's Free Church, where they held a service before striding out, heading by the Lord Provost, to join the throng; the City's sword and mace, silver batons and halberds were all draped in black. The members of the Chamber of Commerce and the Merchants of Edinburgh mustered 300 to take part in the processions. The legal faculties were represented by contingents as numerous, advocates, Writers of the Signet, lawyers and solicitors, each in their own group.

All moved, as if drawn by a magnet, towards Queen Street, where already bands representing the artistic societies, philosophical institutes, antiquarians and geologists had found their way through the gathering crowds and were being hustled into position by the City Clerk. Only the 200-strong band of students—quick to protest then, as now—had objected to their allocated position, and had insisted on forming up between the Obstetrical Society and the College of Surgeons. To Police Inspector Linton fell the task of marshalling the whole contingent into place, and at length the procession moved off at 2.45 p.m., 2,000 people in all.

The elaborate coffin, richly covered in French silk velvet and lavishly decorated with brass knobs, lay on a bier twelve feet in length. Tall black plumes balanced on the heavily draped and fringed canopy, supported by black ornamental pillars. Black tassels, black crêpe, black plumes, black velvet —everypossible mark of respect due to the dead had been paid.

But no worldly trappings could distract attention from the stillness at the heart of it all—a profound silence, perceptible to the watching crowds despite the clattering hooves of the six magnificent horses which bore the hearse creaking and swaying through the hushed streets. A lone carriage followed, its emptiness more poignant to the spectators than the Victorian splendour of the magnificent funeral carriage with its large Belgian horses, white-trousered postilions, mutes and all. Never again would it bear the untidy, uncouth-looking man rattling over the Edinburgh cobbles to his beloved University square.

The cortege moved slowly along Queen Street and turned at right angles into Hanover Street. The curve of Dundas Street lay ahead, dipping downhill towards the river Forth. A solid wall of people lined either side of the streets, the poor of the tenements mingling with their prosperous neighbours from the Georgian squares and crescents. Every inch of standing room was occupied, every window white with faces, every balcony crammed. Higher still, people could even be seen on the steep, sloping roofs, clutching at the chimney stacks.

The long line of mourners wended its serpentine way through the dense crowd of onlookers. Every now and then the sun glittered on the gilt plates on the side of the coffin, throwing it into relief against the dead blackness of the bier. There was no sound from the 80,000 watching people, only the trudging feet of the procession and the subdued hum that goes with a crowd and hangs above it in the air.

Reaching the foot of the hill, the cortege crossed the bridge into Inverleith Row, passing the children of the Ragged Schools drawn up in front of the spectators. Now the crowd lost importance to the trees, which swayed in a gusty wind which muffled the footsteps and swallowed up the subdued hum of people in the mass. Past the Botanic Gardens, then a right turn, and the cemetery was reached. The mile-long procession was all through the gates by four o'clock.

The family burying ground was on a slope. The relatives and friends and the representatives of the scientific bodies gathered above the grave, and the students and the rest of the vast contingent, below. The general public were everywhere, and the Lord Provost with the Town Council took a dignified stance on the catacombs. There was no service, only a pause while a hush settled over the throng, then the pallbearers lowered the coffin into the grave. The sods fell solidly on top. The sky became overcast and it began to rain. As a stream of women slipped forward to lay down wreaths and bunches of flowers around the grave, the vast crowds slowly began to disperse, making their way back up the long slope, beginning to talk quietly among themselves, gradually bringing life back to its normal pace.

Royalty could scarcely have been accorded more honour. Yet on that day, Friday, 13 May 1870, no royal duke had been buried, but a man of humble birth, a citizen of Edinburgh, and a servant of the people. His name was James Young Simpson. Who was this man? What had he done?

CHAPTER I

Bathgate, 1810

ST BARTHOLOMEW'S EVE was a black night for the Protestants of France. A few of the Huguenot families managed to hide from the Catholic swords, and so escape the massacre. Some fled to Holland and some across the water to England. One family called Jervais went farther afield, braved the bleak North Sea and sailed up the Firth of Forth into Lowland Scotland. They landed in Grangemouth, bought a little land nearby and, as they had done in France, worked hard to plough and till the soil. The more aristocratic families in the neighbourhood soon noticed and enjoyed the company of the French emigrants, which eventually led to a mixing of bluer blood into the strain. The Jervais farm was called Baldurdie Mains, and was near the little village of Torphicen, a few miles from the larger town of Bathgate.

By the 1750s the cultured, lively Jervais family were on good terms with their neighbours in the adjoining farm of Slackend. This was owned by Alexander Simpson who was well known in the district, as he practised farriery as well as farming, and was much sought after for his cures. His receipt for a Scabit horse, which was considered very good, was to "take 2 ozs of rock minerals and 2 ozs of the sulphur of ferus and 2 ozs of the flour of Brimstone and a bottle of train oil or as much as will cover him all, and in the course of the 8th day after take winter-green oil along with soap and mustard and wash him all over. Keep him warm in the meantime of the operation!"

Cattle plague, the Murrain, hit the cows of the area in the mid 1770s and everyone looked to Alexander for a cure. His usual potions did nothing to keep the outbreak in check—people blamed the evil eye, and the only cure for that was to bury a cow alive. So Alexander, with the help of his youngest son, dug a shallow pit and pushed in an elderly cow. The son, David, remembered to his last day how the ground heaved after the grave was closed in. A corner of the farm was fenced off as a present to the evil Spirit—or Auld Clootie as she was called; it still remains, a stony, thorny, triangular patch at the edge of a sloping field.

The small farmers of Lowland Scotland were a select breed. They worked hard on their own land, were very independent, asking no one's help, were strong Presbyterians and their boys and girls attended the village school. There they learned their Bible, classics and maths; most farmers had some books on their shelves, the most thumbed being usually the Shorter Catechism and *Scots Worthies*, a collection of biographical sketches of men of the Church—Presbyterian of course.

Alexander Simpson had married an Isabella Grindlay and they lived a peaceful agricultural life on the rich, rolling farm-land of West Lothian, or Linlithgowshire as the county was called then. They believed firmly in the Church, but in the supernatural too. They cured any ailments that befell them in the traditional ways handed down in the folklore of Scotland. Holding a live puppy to the stomach relieved the colic, and white onions and oil, the pangs of childbirth. Blood letting was the usual treatment for anything else.

Alexander and Isabella had four sons, and two of these caused them some trouble. They insisted on setting off to see the wicked world, and had headed south on foot for London. Alexander wrote them a long letter in 1783. It begins abruptly, "David and George, this comes to let you both know that we are all in some mesure of helth at present, blessed he be that gives it. Your mother has had a long sore troubel, but she is a deall better. Your letter befor was like a cure to her but your last made her to trembel." This was referring to the lads' narrow escape from the press gang. "Don't long for riches," advised Alexander, "it sometimes takes the wings of the morn-ing and flies away." As letters only cost 10d, he urged them to write often and added that he would pay their fare home from any port and that they must on no account become involved with the army. The boys came north again a year later.

David was an easy-going, friendly lad, always ready for a joke. As he was the youngest of the four sons, there was no room for him on the farm. Instead, he took to the honourable trade of whisky producing, and set up his own distillery in the nearby

village of Glenmavis. In 1792 he married the daughter of the
neighbouring farm, Mary Jervais. She was quick and sunny,
and had inherited much of her great grandfather's lively French
blood. The distillery prospered, as it must with so much whisky
drunk, and the couple had six children. Then new excise laws
came in, followed by the Peninsular War, and the price of corn
became prohibitive. David tried brewing instead, but could
not make this project work either.

David had learnt to make bread during his wandering days
in the South and now he turned to this as an alternative. He
set up a little shop in Main Street, Bathgate. It was a small
stone house set squint to the road where the post horses of the
Glasgow–Edinburgh coach rang their hooves on the cobbles as
they clattered past.

Bathgate was the market town for the farming community
around. As well as vegetables and corn, the farmers brought
in flax that was grown and dried in the fields sloping towards
the Forth. Most of the people living in Bathgate worked at the
weaving trade, buying the flax and spinning it themselves before
settling down at their looms. The women spun, while the men
of the family sat with their shuttles just inside the front door
which opened onto the main room. The people worked for
themselves, and were independent and intelligent. Those that
were not had either fallen by the wayside or moved to the
mechanical looms being set up on the industrial west-coast
towns, where jobs could be had, if one was prepared to live with
the riff-raff of Ireland flocking out of their own hungry land

Things were going badly in the baker's shop in 1811. The
business was heavily in debt, and, the last straw, there was
another baby on the way. It came early, on 7 July, and the local
doctor, Dawson, was too late to help at the birth, although he
charged a fee of 10/–. Another son was born, the seventh. They
called him James Young.

The family was at hits lowest ebb; the shop had made 8/3 on
the day the new baby was born. This extra mouth to feed forced
Mary up off her bed in a final attempt to keep their heads above
water. She was now forty and, with the difficulties of her confinement safely behind her, she turned her attention to the shop.
She took over the bakery accounts and began to pull things
together. Neighbours commented on the change in fortune that

seemed to coincide with the birth of the seventh son. In a few months the Simpson family moved to a two-storey house across the street.

The yongest baby in a large family has plenty of love. There are many hands for the chores, and someone's arms are always free. Mary was particularly affectionate, and now that the pressure was off and the elder children contributing to the family purse, she had time to sit with the new baby. He has been remembered as a "rosy bairn wi' laughin' mou' and dimpled cheeks".

He was a particularly receptive, forthcoming child with plenty of smiles and a mass of ginger curls on his big head. The world was his friend as he toddled about the house with its front-room shop. The six much elder brothers and one sister drew him out. Partly because of this and partly because of his close contact with his mother, he was ready for school at the age of four. James was small, but square, thickset and sturdy. He had the sort of shape that a mother can never keep neat: one energetic hitch on his part, and waist and shoulders would meet. He was not a restless child, either moving purposefully, or sitting calmly in a corner with a book.

The headmaster of the little school remembered long after that he had called this child "the wise wean" and had noted a lively, alert eye in the rather mature though fat face. Education was considered a privilege in a Scottish home in those days, and each family longed for at least one son to get to university. The Simpsons put their hopes on James. They encouraged him to read rather than help in the shop, although it was his job to ride round the cottages early in the morning on the family pony delivering the newly baked rolls. There was always time for a chat among the weavers, although the shuttle never stopped, and the child was always welcome at the door. Father David was a popular man and the wives and farming folk would linger in the baker's shop to hear him tell a tale, or join him for a whisky in one of the many pubs.

When James was nine, his mother died. The only sister Mary took over the home and the mother's love for her youngest child, and almost filled the gap. Mary held the home together and the Simpson family was, and is, close knit and affectionate. The brothers and father looked for something of their mother in

the young boy, and lavished on him their love and encouragement. He did, in fact, take after his mother: his voice and senti-
mentality, and his gentleness seemed to reflect the Jervais
genes. In Lowland Scotland it was permissible to be different,
and no one laughed at the somewhat studious boy as he wrote
in the flour on the baker's counter instead of parcelling up the
rolls. Everyone agreed that knowledge was more important than
money or position—that is why the minister and the teacher
were the leaders of the community, even though often among
the poorest section.

Uncle George, on the Jervais side, kept one of the local inns.
He was well known for his politeness and for the wealth of his
conversation. He had a large collection of engravings and
knick-knacks, and rubbings that he had made himself. He liked
to wander about old graveyards, peering at tombs, and was
often accompanied on these ramblings by his nephew James.
Together they went all the way to Edinburgh, when the boy
was nine, and spent a long time among the old graves in Grey-
friars Churchyard, just within the old city wall. This was
James's first visit to the capital city. As they approached
Edinburgh from the west, the Pentland hills were a soft green
backdrop to a black skyline of church spires, St Giles Orb, the
bulk of tenement lands, and the Castle, aloof and by itself,
supreme on its rock. It is the same to this day.

The ambition of a bright boy from Bathgate in the nineteenth
century was to become a student at Edinburgh University.
Many of them did, and they enjoyed returning to the old
school in their home town to show off their sophistication and
city ways to the admiring scruffy schoolboys they had left
behind. James Simpson was particularly impressed with the
appearance of his former friend, John Reid, lately returned
from Edinburgh, and he resolved to own a cane like his and to
follow in his shoes. The schoolmaster and the family were as
enthusiastic and they sent James off, at the age of fourteen,
towards the city lights of Edinburgh, to join the University.

CHAPTER II

Edinburgh, 1825

WHEN JAMES VI rode south in 1603 to be King of England as well as the North, Edinburgh lost the Court and all that went with it. The city was even harder hit when Parliament was abolished in 1707. The exodus of the Scottish nobility from the capital was a loss that it could not afford to bear. Vitality and talent, intellect and art, drained south. The city went to sleep. There was an air of gloom and depression throughout Scotland and this national torpor was only temporarily disturbed by the Rebellion of 1715 and the Porteous mob riots of 1736, when two smugglers were condemned to death. At the execution, the mob, who were in sympathy with the victims, attacked the guard. The captain, John Porteous, ordered the guard to fire into the rabble and some of them were killed. He was then tried for murder and sentenced to death. Sir Robert Walpole, Prime Minister at the time weighed up the circumstances, and the captain was reprieved. The people of Edinburgh, however, were incensed. They broke into the guard house, dragged Porteous off to the place of execution and hanged him themselves.

In September 1745 there were a few days of gaiety while Prince Charles was proclaimed king: the fires and lamps were lit in Holyrood and the people flocked to the Cross. For a short time the old glories were revived, but stagnation set in once more.

Tne coronation of George III in 1752 was celebrated with surprising excitement. Cannon fire heralded the coming of the Georgian age and the birth of the New Town of Edinburgh. The great guns of the Castle boomed out, answered by volleys from the warships drawn up off the coast in Leith Roads, and at four o'clock the magistrates and leading citizens went in procession to Parliament House to drink the health of the new king. In the evening the city was illuminated, and fireworks let off from a boat in the Nor' Loch. This had a fine effect on the water, remembered long after the loch disappeared from the Edinburgh scene.

Edinburgh till then had been a medieval city. The town was built on a ridge running from the Castle on its high rock down to Holyrood Palace at the foot of the Salisbury Crags. The High Street lay down this ridge, with a series of wynds and closes descending on either side. To the north, green fields, and to the south, the parklands of the monasteries of Black and Grey Friars. The people huddled together, living on top of each other safe behind the city walls. A coach left from Glasgow only twice a week. Communication with the South was practically non-existent, although the *Caledonian Mercury* did advertise on Thursday, 9 May 1734 that "a coach would set out towards the end of the week for London". It was to go faster than any other and would take only nine days. This was possible by having eighty horses staged along the way.

Various enlightened people had considered enlarging the town, but it was not until 1767 that an act was passed allowing the city to breach the walls and overflow on to the green fields that spread northwards down towards the Firth of Forth. The papers of the day carried advertisements inviting architects to submit plans for the laying out of a new town. Those of James Craig were successful and the pattern of streets and squares of the Edinburgh that we know began to take shape. The wondering eyes of the older inhabitants saw their Nor' Loch drained at the foot of the Castle rock and a great line of communication thrown across the gully dividing the Old and New Towns. In the next thirty-seven years, £3,000,000 were spent on building. George Drummond, the Lord Provost, and his City fathers showed considerable width of vision in risking such a tremendous sum of money, for the community was by no means wealthy.

The activity was now fantastic. As the building went on, the earth excavated from the houses in the New Town was thrown into the Nor' Loch and the Mound began to take shape. The physicians now laid the foundation stone of their new hall in George Street and the Royal Dispensary opened its doors. In 1788, with a great Masonic procession, the foundation stone was laid for Robert Adam's elegant University Building on the South Bridge, and 30,000 people were interested enough to stand and watch. Little did they know that the £32,000 allocated was not enough and that the work would not be completed until 1815.

This was a splendid era of progress; and, as always, one circle of vigour and enthusiasm sparked off others. There was now a class in Edinburgh which did not have to devote all its energies to a battle for existence, and as the stress of living became less people were able to devote time and money to leisure pursuits: the Bruntsfield Golf Club was founded in 1761, and the Nicolson Street Riding Academy in 1764. There were enough people interested in antiquities to found a society in 1783 and enough horse owners to form a Caledonian Hunt in 1778.

By the end of the eighteenth century, 81,865 people lived in Edinburgh. The post still took sixty hours to reach London, but the influence of the more gracious South was making itself felt. The New Town was the place to live. The aristocratic families of Scotland began to take an interest in law and commerce, and the growing prosperity drew the best young minds of the generation to the Scottish capital, stemming the inevitable drift of ability south. In fact there was a reversal, and intellectual London began to regard Edinburgh as a centre of culture. The Napoleonic wars prevented writers and artists from flocking across the Channel to the great centres on the Continent. Naismith stayed at home to paint the Scottish scene, Raeburn to take the portraits of a generation of Scottish worthies. William Playfair was now making his mark on the architectural scene, his straight Grecian lines appearing all over the city.

This gay, debonair, social yet cultured life in Edinburgh reached its peak in the mid 1820s. Lord Cockburn and Lord Jeffries were in the thick of it. So also was Sir Walter Scott. This was a city of theology and law, a university city where town and gown mixed freely. Its learning and politics, together with its romantic history won Edinburgh particular renown. The Rev. Sydney Smith found Edinburgh "energetic and un-fragrant", but he was prepared to spend "five years in discussing metaphysics and medicine in that garret of the Earth, that knuckle end of England, that land of Calvin, oatcakes and sulphur". A concentration of literary young men had flourished in Edinburgh since the turn of the century. In 1803 Thomas Jeffries and his friends inspired the publication of the *Edinburgh Review* with Sydney Smith as the first editor. The paper was a happy relationship between English and Scottish intellect and the literary Scot now had a chance to be taken seriously by the London set. Each new number was looked upon as an event in the articulate world. Despite its English editor, the paper was peculiarly imbued with the spirit of Edinburgh, with articles on poetry, politics and theology, written at a conversational level, directed at a public interested, without being experts, in a world of culture, and ready to be amused by satire and wit. The writers were amateurs, so the articles were written in the common conversational tongue. It became the habit in Edinburgh for any reasonably educated man to put down his opinions in print, to publish all his ideas and theories, often publicly to criticise the works of his fellows. Thus began a tradition inherited by James Y. Simpson and his colleagues. The *Scotsman* joined the *Edinburgh Review* in January 1817. A solicitor, William Ritchie, was the most active of the three founders. He joined the project to float the weekly paper because he could find no other journal that would print his criticism on the management of the Edinburgh Royal Infirmary! This liberal paper signified the freedom of the press. The sparkling and scandalous articles on these papers were discussed with great enthusiasm at the fashionable evening parties held in George Square and the big houses in the crescents of the New Town. Here life was gayer than ever. Elizabeth Grant of Rothiemurchus tells us in her *Memoirs of a Highland Lady* that the quadrilles had come into vogue but were much frowned on by the "old fashioned respectables" who felt that they were far too intimate and informal, and the conversations much too free. Lord Cockburn gives a clear picture of social and articulate Edinburgh with its clubs and debating societies, yet he does not neglect the other side of the scene.

Life for the poor in the Old Town of Edinburgh was as grim as it had been five generations earlier. In 1795 11,000 people were fed by charity in Edinburgh (the food was cooked on "Count Romford's", a new stove that cut down the clouds of black smoke that up till now had added to the grime and misery of the poor). In 1816 the situation was even worse: according to

Lord Cockburn "This year closed bitterly for the poor. There never had been so many people destitute at one time." The Highland Clearances were blamed for the influx of people to the towns, but a high proportion were not Highlanders, but Irish. They arrived in Glasgow by the thousands and drifted east. A Mr Robert Johnstone wrote to the press of his idea of using bands of these destitute poor "to make roads round the Calton Hill, which paths embrace views almost unrivalled in the world—also a new line of road through Holyrood Park and in levelling Bruntsfield Links—part of the common good of Edinburgh". This scheme was put into effect, and the whins and gorse bushes were cleared from the Meadows and the old quarries tidied up. £10,000 was spent on paving roads and cobbling new streets, the Prince Regent donating £1,000 to pay for a path along the foot of the Salisbury Crag. The citizens were delighted, particularly with the view west from the new Regent Road around Colton Hill.

However, Lord Cockburn "had only begun to perceive its importance when its interception by the North Bridge Buildings raised our indignation and we thought that the magistrates who allowed them to be set agoing in silence had betrayed us. We were therefore very angry and had recourse to another of these new things called public meetings which we were beginning to feel the power of." But, writes Cockburn, "we lost one thousand pounds and the buildings stand". But much good was done by the clamour. Attention was called, nearly for the first time, to the duty of maintaining the beauty of Edinburgh. The people were involved with their town planning and administration and what happened in it to an extent not seen today, and they were prepared to take the law into their own hands if necessary. There was, for instance, the "shocking affair" of the execution of Robert Johnstone. The new Calton gaol had just been built, when Johnstone, aged twenty-three, was convicted of highway robbery and condemned to execution on 30 December. This being the first execution after the removal of the old gaol, a temporary scaffold had been erected with its gibbet resting on the wall of St Giles. But it was put up in a hurry and when the drop fell, the culprit was left on his toes. The mob was horrified, not at the execution but at the mismanagement of it! They stoned the magistrates and police, cut down the victim, revived him and carried him off. However the Provost won the day. He called in the troops who waylaid the mob, dragged back young Johnstone, and he was successfully hanged.

This then was the Edinburgh in which James Young Simpson found himself in 1825; a country lad of fourteen, in his brother's corduroy suit—"thick set, fat, sonsy, callant, a wide face with dimples on his cheeks in a particularly large head." He remembered later that he felt "very very young and very solitary, very poor and almost friendless" as he unpacked his bag in No. 1 Adam Street, Stockbridge, where he was to pay 3/– per week for digs. Dr McArthur, who had taught for a while at the Bathgate School, let out the top floor of this old tenement house and already had another local lad, Simpson's old schoolmate, John Reid, as a boarder when James moved in.

It was quite common for boys to come to university at an age when they would now be in their first years at secondary school. It was also common for the boys to be poor. Lads from the parish schools came to town with a few books and a sack of meal and a few shillings to see them through the term. The sons of the country gentry and the professional men were there too, with a smattering from England putting in a few years before going on to Oxbridge. Most of the boys, however, were from Edinburgh itself, quicker-witted and more on the spot, as city boys are to this day. The remarkable thing about the Scottish universities was the large part they played in life of the nation. They were cheap and there was no entrance examination, but the young Scots were all serious students for there were very few whose future did not depend on their work.

For generations the great hopes of a Scottish working-class family had been to have one son clever enough to enter the Ministry. Every sacrifice was worth making for this ultimate goal. The result was that education was almost entirely academic. Latin was essential. It was international, and in the older days had been used conversationally among the travelling scholars of the British as well as Continental universities. Philosophy was the subject most sought after, divided into Metaphysics, logic and humanity. Subjects such as literature, geology or modern languages were considered inferior—below the notice of the really clever boy.

Following the Scottish universities' system, Simpson enrolled by taking out his first "class tickets" in Junior Greek and Humanity which cost him £3 each. These were the days when the character of the professor had a direct influence on the student—it really mattered who filled the chair. The Professor of Humanity at Edinburgh University at this time was the famous James Pillans, an ex-headmaster of the High School, where he had made his mark on many a lad now striding into the Edinburgh scene. Pillans believed that a young mind must be trained to "accuracy, endurance and depth, and exercised with perseverance on a few subjects only" and "what better than Latin or Greek for strengthening the memory, attention, imagination and judgement? Also useful at infusing an accurate and ready use of the English language . . . or as indispensable as the ground work for learning a foreign modern tongue." That Simpson ultimately proved this point beyond doubt we shall see. Pillans' interest in the Arts was far wider than the study of classical subjects warranted and he was responsible for an exhibition in Edinburgh in 1822 of watercolours of Grecian scenery, with appropriate classical quotations, much admired by Lord Cockburn and the intelligentsia of the town.

Among the bevy of young lads facing Pillans in 1825 he singled out the chubby-cheeked Simpson, not because of any scholastic merit but for his lively eye and enthusiastic air—his essays "contained vigorous thinking and a grace of style seldom met with" in a boy of fifteen. Simpson had been outstandingly clever at Bathgate but had the rude shock of being very much an "also ran" at Edinburgh. Pillans apparently appreciated the inadequacies of his parochial education and, in spite of very average class marks, urged him to compete for the Stewart Bursary at the beginning of his second year.

Scottish universities were fortunately well supplied with these small open scholarships left by those who valued education but had often seen none themselves. This one was for £10, tenable for three years and open to boys called Stewart or Simpson, who were tested on their Latin Prose. Nothing is known of the competition for the bursary, but Simpson won it, and this seemed to spur him on. "Tolerably good" was still the usual remark written in the margin of his returned work—"Very bad", however, on an essay for Professor Dunbar who held the chair in Greek.

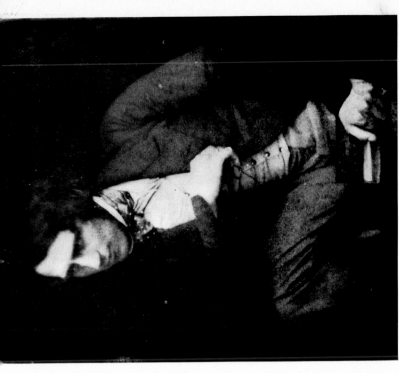

The new professor, 29 years old. Early calyotype by D. O. Hill. Considered to be Simpson by the National Portrait Gallery of Scotland

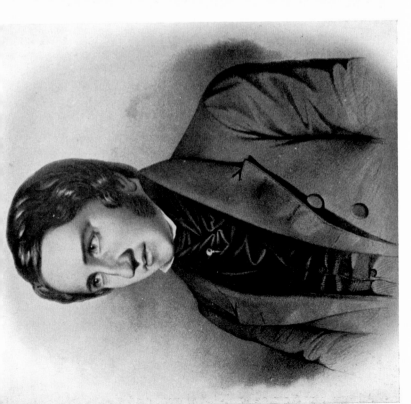

The young doctor

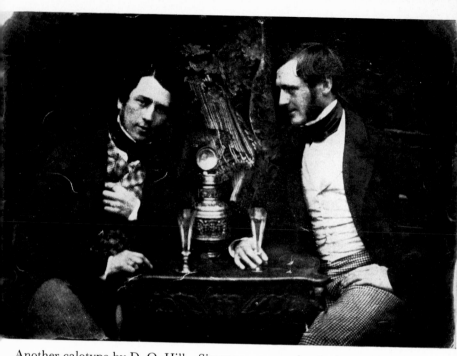

Another calotype by D. O. Hill—Simpson presumed to be in tartan waistcoat

My Dear Miss Grindlay

Have you got 7½ᵈ to spare to the postman. I have got half an hour to spare till my coffee is ready, & intend patriotically to devote it to the good of my country's exchequer by fining you the laid sums for your wilful negligence & dead, perverse silence. In lieu of your 7½ᵈ I give you three facts—(price 2½ each) 'dear'- very!

1. I have at last taken the house round the corner! £ - - - - 2½

2. I have hired a Housekeeper from Dublin!! - - .. - 2½

3. Miss P—k is married at last to a sailor!!! - .. - 2½

£ - n - 7½

What do you think of your bargain?—

Yours very faithfully

J Y Simpson. —

A letter from Simpson to his lady love, Miss Grindley

James was prepared to work hard at his classics and he led a strictly disciplined life. He and the other two boys in the lodging house would clamber up the dark stair after their classes had finished at 3.00 p.m., dip their finnan haddies in boiling water, push their plates out of the way and spread their books over the table. MacArthur held sway in that particular garret and John Reid and Simpson did as he told them. He got them up at crack of dawn for a few hours study before their first class at 8.00 a.m. then kept them working far into the night. Mac-Arthur wrote to Simpson's brother, Sandy, "I can now do with four hours sleep, John Reid can do with six but I have not been able to break in James yet." Simpson's carefully kept account book of this year has the entry "Book on Early Rising 9½d". It must have been a worthwhile investment, for in 1842 he was to tell his students in their graduation address, "It has been calculated that the simple difference between rising at 6 and at 9 o'clock in the morning for the expanse of 40 years is nearly equivalent to the addition of 15 years to a man's life." He certainly carried out this theory himself. He also at this time spent 9d on *The Economy of Human Life* and in true Presbyterian tradition copied out on the fly leaf of his notebook, "Let not thy recreations be expensive lest the pain of purchasing them exceed the pleasures thou hast in their enjoyment." At this age he was certainly counting his pennies and each carefully completed account book was sent home for brother Sandy to scrutinise. That this was not quite true to character is borne out by stories of his carelessness with money at a later date. For instance, it is related that, spending the night in a patient's draughty bedroom, Simpson stuffed the rattling window with a bank note and completely forgot to retrieve it the following morning!

John Reid, Simpson's fellow lodger in Adam Street, was studying medicine, and was particularly interested in anatomy, a subject which excited much interest in the young James, and in Edinburgh in general. In 1826 the infamous Dr Knox was still at the helm, although the Professor of Anatomy was actually Alexander Munro. Knox's lectures in anatomy were so clear and pithy that at one time his classes were attended by more than 500 young men—not only students of medicine but of literature, law and classics too—and he gave his daily lecture three times over, often consecutively. This success, however, proved to be a problem as Knox was determined that his pupils should have the best practical instruction. Knox's advertisement for the anatomy course stated that "each of these courses" will comprise a full Demonstration on Fresh Anatomical subjects". This meant that Knox was one of the best customers of the resurrectionists who were the only source of bodies for the dissection table. This trade had been going on for well over 100 years and was carried out with great boldness in Edinburgh. A dark winter's evening was chosen for the deed of body snatching, between six and eight o'clock. A hole was dug at the head end of the coffin, the earth being carefully laid on a canvas sheet so that the smooth uniformity of the grass was not spoilt. Wooden dagger-shaped diggers were used so as to prevent the clink of spade on stone. Two broad iron hooks were then pushed under the lid of the coffin; a strong yank on the attached rope broke off enough of the lid for access to the body which was dragged out through the hole. The shrouds were carefully removed and buried again with great care. The body was pushed into a sack and the surface of the ground carefully restored to its original condition. This was easy as the sods of a newly dug grave always looked disturbed. The whole job could be completed in an hour even though the grave was six feet deep. Several men worked together and there was no difficulty in swinging the loaded sack over the graveyard wall. Once in the street, the resurrectionist was safe: there was nothing omnious in a figure hurrying along so early in the evening with a sack on his back.

As long as there were only two lecturers on anatomy in Edinburgh, resurrectioning went on smoothly, each man having his own territory on which the other did not encroach. However, when a third lecturer entered the field and ignored these arrangements, trouble arose among the rival parties. A lookout man would wait on the churchyard wall, ready to stake a claim at the first approach of the rivals by dropping down and standing astride the grave. John Reid and his friends, with a love of adventure, often took part in the affrays which then ensured. Because of the rows between the parties and the rashness that came about as a result, the town Authorities felt obliged to take some steps and a stricter watch was established. Resurrectioning became a riskier undertaking. The public, now better informed, began to erect the iron cages still to be seen in the older church-yards in Edinburgh, over many a family grave, and the anatomists found that there were not enough bodies to go around. The price for a clrpse rose to £20 and the temptation to get one must have been great. There now arose in Edinburgh, as there had been in London for some time, a gang of pro-fessional body snatchers, usually the greatest scoundrels in the community. The step between stealing the dead and murdering the living was small. This conclusion was reached by Mr Burke and his mistress, Helen or Mary M'Dougal, who joined partner-ship with a Mr Hare and his wife. They set up a lodging house to which they lured their victims. They plied them with drink and then suffocated them so that the body showed no trace of violence. They were so successful that they grew careless and a visitor noticed a body beneath Burke's bed. It was carried by Burke to the anatomy department of Dr Knox early next morning in a tea chest, but the alarm had been raised, and the body was claimed by legal authority before Knox or his students set eyes on it. Dr Robert Christison, afterwards a great friend of Simpson's, was called in by the police to conduct the inspection of this body and his report states,

> The subject was a woman about middle age, well nourished, and without a trace of disease in any organ. The body presented the signs of death by asphyxia—vague—as there were no external marks about the neck or face to indicate how her respiration had been obstructed. There was injury to the cervical spine which had been caused soon after death while the body was warm. There were bruises on the limbs occasioned not long before death and might have been caused by blows or kicks . . . every particular appearance we observed was consistent with the idea of death by suffocation . . . smothering and not strangling was the manner of it.

The city and country generally were thrown into a state of horror by the exposure of what were called "the West Port murders" and Burke and Hare were looked upon as monsters. People's attention then turned to Dr Knox who had presumably turned a blind eye on Burke's and Hare's activities. The

B

bodies were delivered to him warm and flexible and obviously had never been under the ground. However, it was a stroke of sheer bad luck that Burke and Hare delivered this particular body to Knox and not one of the other anatomists in the town, all of whom they also supplied from time to time, receiving from £7. 10s. od. to £10 for each full sack. The Edinburgh citizens were outraged, and Knox was made the scapegoat of the entire resurrectionist affair. His colleagues, instead of backing him up, assumed an attitude of selfrighteous indignation, and Knox's only champions were to be his students.

The press kept the pot boiling for the six weeks that elapsed before the trial, which was scheduled to begin on Christmas Eve. Tremendous public interest was aroused, and the streets between Calton Gaol and the court house in Parliament Close was packed when the day arrived. The doors of the court were opened at nine o'clock, and, according to the *Courant* were instantly filled to suffocation point. Hare turned King's Evidence, leaving Burke and M'Dougal to be tried for a single murder, that of the old woman. But as the story unfolded it became clear that about sixteen murdered bodies were involved; luckily for M'Dougal, Henry Cockburn was her counsel, and his eloquence won her her life. She was set free within twenty-four hours, and disappeared from the scene. Burke, however, was proved guilty and 20,000 spectators were reported in the *Courant* to have gathered to witness his execution. Seats in all the windows of the old houses overlooking the scaffold had been sold to fashionable Edinburgh for from 5 to 25 shillings. Punctually at 8.00 a.m. on 28 January 18■■ Burke appeared, to be greeted with a fantastic roar. He died fifteen minutes later with the crowd yelling and shouting with excitement.

The next day the body was carried to the University to be dissected (ironically enough by Professor Munro), and 24,000 people are reported to have filed past as it lay spread out on the dissecting slab. The skeleton now hangs in the Edinburgh Royal College of Surgeons' Museum, so presumably the citizens of Edinburgh feel Burke has still not paid for his sins.

Burke's death did not satisfy the people of the city, and when they realised that no other pound of flesh was to be legally extracted over the affair, they took the law into their own hands. A furious mob gathered together on the night of 12

February and, carrying a guy of Knox, marched to his house in Arniston Place in the Newington district of the town. They hung this effigy on a tree and tried to set it alight. A cold damp wind put out the flames, so the mob tore their guy to pieces instead, then smashed the windows and were about to sack the house when the police arrived. Knox had meanwhile walked out of his back door. He refused to be intimidated by this mass violence, and, in spite of pickets about his lecture theatre, never missed a class. This so impressed the students that they collected money for a presentation golden vase as a token of their respect. Simpson and John Reid contributed 2/6 each.

Henry Cockburn also kept his admiration for Knox and wrote in his journal, "Our anatomists were spotlessly correct and Knox the most correct of them all." He adds the last words of the story of the affair,

> Except that he murdered, Burke was a sensible, and what might be called a respectable man; not at all ferocious in his general manner, sober, correct in all his other habits and kind to his relations. Though not regularly married, Mary M'Dougal was his wife; and when the jury came in with the verdict convicting him, but aquitting her, his remark was . . . "Well, thank God your safe".

However, most influential people in Edinburgh were against Knox, including Sir Walter Scott and the editors of the *Scotsman* and *Courant* newspapers, along with Christopher North, now Professor of Moral Philosophy. The latter attacked Knox in a long article in *Blackbwoods Magazine*.

Eventually Knox gave up the struggle, and in 1842 left Edinburgh, abandoning, at thirty-six, his life's work. He relied on journalism and lecturing for an income for the next twenty years, travelling about the country entertaining an audience on the elastic subject, "Races of Men". He had become intrigued by the racial differences between the Highland Celtic Scot and the Lowlander, and his interest in ethnology had increased with his sojourn in Africa, and contact with the black races of the Cape. When a tribe of Ojibway Indians created a sensation in London in 1839, Knox studied them closely and added the Red Indian to his lecture repertoire. Knox had no definite job until 1856 when he was appointed Pathological Anatomist to the pioneer cancer hospital in London. Just as his career seemed to be improving, he died of heart disease, on 20 December 1862. His tragic life story, revealing Edinburgh's intolerance, jealousy persecution and the influence that current public opinion could bring to bear, is an important factor in considering the background of any medical man of those times.

We must go back to the heyday of Knox, however, as it was his inspired teaching and infectious enthusiasm that seemed first to have interested Simpson in the subject of medicine. Anatomical sketches and snippets of information that he had picked up from Knox mingled with Latin syntax and Greek grammar in the young student's notebooks. In one of them he records that a single Kaffir had once polished off a band of British soldiers by knowing the exact spot in which to plunge his knife so that it struck the main artery of the neck, which resulted in the victim falling without uttering even a groan.

Simpson's fellow lodgers, Reid and MacArthur, further fostered this casual interest in medicine, and in 1827 Simpson enrollled as a medical student without bothering to complete his arts course.

CHAPTER III

The Medical Student

THE TEACHING OF medicine in 1827 was somewhat haphazard. The regulations for taking the degree were that in certain subjects students had to take out class tickets and attend the professor's course of lectures, but they only needed to put in an appearance at a sufficient number in order to obtain the necessary certificate; the real study of the subject was made outside the university walls. Students decided themselves which of the many extramural or private classes to attend and which surgeons, physicians and anatomists to follow. They then presented themselves for examination when they felt ready.

Knox, as we have seen, held the field in anatomy, Abercrombie and Gregory were the leading physicians. Personality and character drew students as much as ability and Dr Gregory filled his classes on this account. He had taught his theories for forty-one years so that a large part of the country and colonies were doctored by his methods, and Gregory's Mixture was pushed down the throats of the population by the gallon. Gregory's Powder is still to be seen in little shops in the West of Scotland; magnesia, rhubarb and ginger are its main constituents.

Gregorian physic—"free blood letting, cold affusion, brisk purging, frequent blisters, the nauseating action of tartar emetic"—had ruled medical practice for many years. No wonder that the more enlightened students of Simpson's era began to wonder if there was not some alternative, and dabbling in homeopathy came into vogue. Simpson's notes on the "Practice of Physic" deal mainly with the treating of fever—the cure, of course, being the letting of blood. The average physician of the early Victorian age was armed with a jar of sticky black leeches and a mania for putting them to work. Dr Gregory was a determined, pugnacious man. He carried a cane, always held over one shoulder ready for action. To the delight of his students he once brought it to bear on the current Professor of Midwifery

Dr Hamilton. £100 was eventually paid in damages, which, said Dr Gregory, 'he 'would pay all over again for another opportunity of thrashing the little obstetrician".

These were stirring times in Edinburgh medical circles and the arguments and strife must have made an indelible impression on the students as they crowded into the classroom and heard the learned professors berating each other—not only in words. The lecturers' living depended on the size of attendnace at their class which perhaps explains the hot tempers and everreadiness to be at each other's throats.

Rivalry was even stronger among the surgeons. Robert Liston was pre-eminent in the surgical field in Edinburgh. His extramural class had great attraction for the students. He was a colourful character, operating with flourish, full of dash and daring. He held the record for speed at amputations, and patients flocked to him, preparing themselves up for one quick agonising slash with Liston's knife in place of the slower and more painstaking methods of the other leading surgeon on the horizon, James Syme, Liston's third cousin.

The surgeons of these times kept an old blood-stained coat for operating, with a bunch of silk threads hanging from a buttonhole ready for tying round a gushing artery. The industrial age had begun and was bringing into the hospitals the horrifying results of accidents caused by men, children, women and machines working together. Mangled and fractured limbs were invariably amputated, with a mortality rate of 40 per cent. Patients did not often die from the rigours of the actual operation, but from subsequent infections in the wound left by the surgeon's knife. The smell of gangrene and decay in the surgical wards was, according to a later note of Simpson's, "even worse for a medical student to become accustomed to than any scene during the operation itself".

The heroism of the patient was matched by the heroics of the surgeon, who had to be brutally strong, yet agile and delicate at the same time. Robert Liston had these attributes in a remarkable degree. He was a big, rough-hewn man with a quick temper and a scathing tongue, yet his patients liked him and knew that his heart was in his work.

Liston disapproved of the running of Edinburgh Royal Infirmary, and did not hesitate to say so. This resulted in much public controversy and accusation, and he frequently had to defend himself at the Medical Society and in the press.

The students who had chosen to attend Liston's course of lectures held him in high esteem, and Simpson was among them. His lecture notes for the other professors have queries and question-marks in the margin, but those from Liston have been taken down without comment.

Liston needed bodies for showing the students his methods, and so, like Knox, he was also involved with the resurrectionists. Students vied with each other to help, and no wonder, as the cost of anatomical subjects legally procured was prohibitive to those such as Simpson, on a stipend of £10 a year. In Simpson's notebook, in 1827, he has written, "Bones of the leg—£1".

Yet knowledge of anatomy was vitally important to a surgeon who had to work fast, before his patient died from the pain. Simpson wrote with admiration that Liston "opperated with such speed that the sound of sawing seemed to succeed immediately the first flash of the knife". Operations were measured in seconds, and if a student turned his head, he would often find that he had missed just what he had determined to see. If Liston wanted to use both hands, he was said to save time by holding the knife in his mouth, a habit apparently followed by Edinburgh butchers when separating joints of meat at high speed. Liston was an innovator and taught his students never to be at a loss. Simpson was there among a large crowd, when Liston

had amputated a leg for extensive necrosis and chronic disease of its bones. The patient was feeble, and yet, after securing many vessels, haemorrhage was still abundant from the cut surfaces. More vessels were secured, but the bleeding continued and Professor Russell, who was assisting him, became alarmed lest the patient should sink on the table. At this moment it was discovered that the blood oozed from an enlarged vessel in the substance of the bone. There was a panic of a few seconds, and everyone whispered, what was to be done? Liston immediately sliced off a piece of wood from the operating table with his large amputating knife, and rapidly formed it into a plug, which he thrust into the mouth of the bleeding vessel. The haemorrhage ceased immediately, and the patient recovered.

Students had to obtain certificates of ability from their lecturers at the end of each term, and Liston wrote of Simpson, "He has been a most diligent and attentive student of surgery, he has attended his lectures and examinations with exemplary regularity, and that from his habits of attention I am convinced that he will become a well informed and excellent practitioner."

The medical student's life was full of drama. On an operating day the students would jostle each other as they crowded into the corridor of the Royal Infirmary, and up the stair of the hospital to see if there was a new notice pinned on the board announcing any major operations by the leading surgeon. In the operating room they would talk constantly as they stood crushed into the space allocated to them behind a wooden bar. The patient would be dragged screaming from the ward and held down by grim force on the wooden operating table until the leather belts were buckled tightly across his squirming body and writhing limbs. No wonder speed was the greatest attribute that a surgeon could offer!

The students would watch, but "Don't think them heartless", wrote Dr John Brown in his heartrending story, *Rab and his Friends*, where Ailie, the shepherd's wife, has her breast amputated by James Syme. "They are neither better nor worse than you or I; they get over their professional horrors, and into their proper work; and in them pity, as an emotion, ending in itself or at best in tears and a long drawn breath, lessens,—while pity, as a motive, is quickened, and gains power and purpose. It is well for poor human nature that it is so."

The patients in the hospital wards would be from the Old Town; anyone of standing would summon the surgeon to his own house, and be nursed in his own bed. The poor of Edinburgh at his time were often new to the town. Irish labourers, soldiers back from the Napoleonic wars with nowhere else to go, weavers from the Lothian villages whose work was now being superseded by the big looms in the new-fangled factories of the west coast, and crofters from the glens—all unable to make a living in their own surroundings. Gaelic in fact was often the language of the hospital wards. These people tended, even more than the rest of the community, to look for medical attention only as a last resort, when radical surgery was the all that could be offered for a cure.

During Simpson's term with Liston, a woman from the Highlands who was staying with her daughter in the poor Canongate part of old Edinburgh, was brought into the Infirmary. The students read about her as they gathered round the notice board to see if Liston was carrying out any interesting operations that day. "Amputation of the breast", stated the slip of paper. The technique for this procedure was to lift up the soft tissue by an instrument resembling a bill hook, enabling the surgeon to sweep round the mass with his knife, in two clean cuts.

Simpson was as keen to see this operation as the rest of the students. He had watched others, with an uninvolved interest. This time, however, the old woman in the centre of the stage, with all the male eyes focussing on her, stirred some inner cell in Simpson's mind. He could not bear to see her horrified face as Liston picked up his knife in one hand and gripped her with the other. He turned away, pushed through the crowd of young men and left the room. He hurried out of the hospital gate and up the hill to Parliament Square, where he burst into the imposing building and asked where he could enrol as a clerk, declaring in an agitated voice that he wanted to study law.

This episode was described by Simpson at a much later date. He recollected that he asked himself at that moment, "Can nothing be done to make operations less painful?" He was not really interested in law, and the following day he rejoined his fellow students in the Infirmary.

Medical students have always buried their emotions. Suddenly face to face with raw broken bodies, they have had to force themselves to hide behind a façade of rowdy living, pretending that they do not care, to avoid drowning in a sea of compassion. In Simpson's day, the students went to the ale houses of the Canongate to forget the screams from the hospital wards. They would edge through the bustle fringing the street, push past the carters whose horses champed on the cobbles, step round the water pitchers dumped down by the carriers at the open doors and over the carefully collected bundles of sticks belonging to the faggot sellers. The herds of people cramped into the limited area of the Old Town lived their lives in the streets. There was no room in the dank rabbit warrens of the tenement buildings to do anything but huddle up and sleep. Sir Walter Scott's *Chronicles of the Canongate* describes this life as accurately as a photograph. A poem Simpson wrote during hks student days gives an impression of the atmosphere of gloom pervading the Old Town:

> Our tav'rin bells rang, for the night cloud had lowered,
> And the police night-watch through the city gave roam
> And thousands had sunk from the streets overpowered,
> The flush to get drunk and the poor to get home.

So children played outside, darting through the throng, whizzing barrel hoops, or clearing a space for peevers. Above their high pitched shrieks could be heard the screeching of the garrulous, quarrelsome women as they yelled at each other from either side of the broad road, shawls drawn across their thin shoulders, or hurled greetings and abuse from the high windows of the tall Lands.

Up a stair or through at the back, past the crowds, each tavern would have a few "houffs", private dens habitually filled by a particular group of lawyers, artists or students. The medical students, clutching piles of hard-backed books of painstakingly copied notes, would burst in, loud and high spirited. Simpson was always well to the fore, talking loudly and singing rollicking beery songs. He was a prominent figure in those days, and contemporary diarists often mention his name. Contacts he made at this time he kept for life, and in his own notes to later students, mention of those tavern gatherings often crop up.

According to Simpson it was at one of the taverns that he met the artist who stimulated his interest in drawing and introduced him to Edinburgh's artistic set. Drawing from life was in vogue at the time; the draped figures of the late eighteenth and early nineteenth centuries were making way for more accurate forms. Simspon's advice was aked by his artist friends. He was very short of money, and suddenly he found a way to supplement his £10 bursary and the allowance sent in from Bathgate by his family. He gave classes in anatomical drawing. Precise, delicately shaded pencil sketches of hands and arms, muscles and sinews, filled any spaces in his notebooks at this time. This attention to detail stood him in great stead in later life when he became interested in archaeology; it may also have played a part in his practical approach to obstetrics—for example, in his observation of the shape and size of a baby's head in relation to the mother's pelvis.

There was much to talk about in Edinburgh between 1824 and '29 as the men gathered over the mugs of ale. It was a time of thinking and doing and being involved. Ideas were carried through, like Mr Sadler ascending in a balloon from Heriots Hospital. Great crowds collected to see him and his friend Mr Campbell set off. "The aeronauts crossed the Firth of Forth and landed near Leven in Fife. after a voyage of 2 hours". In the same year Sir Walter Scott was chairman at a public meeting to consider a monument to James Watt. Over 2,000 people attended! Professor Pillans and Henry Cockburn wanted one in Edinburgh, as the disadvantages of the long journey to London were so great. Sir Walter, though, pointed out that since no man had done so much to bring London nearer to Edinburgh as James Watt, London was the place. The audience refused to leave the meeting until Scott agreed to change his mind.

Public meetings were constantly being held in connection with town planning. Rumour had it that building was to commence in the open valley between Old and New Town, and also on the grassy banks between Queen Street and Heriot Row. Lord Cockburn issued pamphlets urging the inhabitants to take action "to preserve the city from destruction".

Whigs and Tories had their support among the 2,200 students at the University in 1826. Representation of the city in Parliament was one of the points at issue. The Reform Bill was also coming up, and protest marches, public meetings and letters to the press came thick and fast. The Lord Advocate, Sir William Rae, was to say in the House of Commons that Scots "could never be trusted with popular election because they never could assemble without bloodshed". Sir Charles Forbes, on the same issue, testified that the Scots "were so ignorant that they did not know what 'reform' or 'representative' meant". The Duke of Buccleuch jumped to his feet and said that the people were desperately interested in the Bill, but it was because they thought it would give them free whisky!

Abolition of slavery was much discussed and Simpson's name appears on a petition in 1829. He attended a meeting in the Assembly Rooms, George Street, at which Dr Andrew

Thomson, the minister of a city church who had already made himself known by outspoken condemnation of the Government and Town Council, spoke again, demanding the immediate freeing of 800,000 slaves. Simpson was very moved by Thomson's speech and quoted from it at a later date.

In speaking of slavery Thomson said, "You may white-wash the sepulchre—you may put upon it every ornament that fancy can suggest—you may cover it over with all the flowers and evergreens that the garden or the fields can furnish, so that it will appear beautiful outwardly unto men. But it is a sepulchre still—full of dead mens' bones and of all uncleaness. Disguise slavery as you will . . . but it is a bitter bitter draught." The Caribbean Islands and the Guianas, where these slaves were working became of great interest to Simpson. He urged his friends to buy shares in property in Tobago and later did himself, and he carried on a vast correspondence with managers and ministers and ship's captains about the ways and means of the local inhabitants: how the Indians took to the African slaves; what sort of snakes lived among the sugar cane; and what was the best way to treat the cane in order to obtain the ultimate sweetness. He asked for samples of sugar and rum, and was always suggesting improvements in the machinery.

Too many people were speculating abroad, and the "Joint Stock Mania", as Cockburn calls it, resulted in disaster. The newspapers carried advertisements and recommendations for every conceivable company. "The schemes were so numerous, that after exhausting every subject to which they could be applied, there was actually a joint stock company instituted for the purpose of organising such companies. Not one honest penny was made out of all this villany and folly," says Lord Cockburn. "The loss was enormous." The Government decided to stop the circulation of Scots £1 notes, and Cockburn wrote,, "Whether this was wise or not, there can be no doubt that the matter was taken up by the government, in a narrow, ignorant, exclusively English spirit. This country was instantly in a blaze from one end to the other. I never saw Scotland unanimous before. It was really refreshing to see the spirit with which the whole land rose as one man. Even the Tories were for a season reconciled to resistance and public meetings."

Such were the current topics and happenings discussed by

students in the alehouses of Edinburgh. When not in the taverns they turned to the country side, for they were lucky in their surroundings. They could amble in the Meadows, or scramble up Arthur's Seat, as freely in 1828 as today. Simpson and Reid particularly enjoyed the southern slopes of Arthur's Seat which drift down to the edge of Duddingston Loch. Otters were to be found there in Simpson's day and the odd badger. Dusky coots and swans lived there, only moving on when the loch was completely frozen and no open water left. Wild duck, teal and water hens nested in the reeds. Pike, perch and eels slithered about below.

The inhabitants of Edinburgh made the most of the winter which swept in on the biting north wind. As soon as the loch froze, skaters flocked out of the town. A contemporary describes a January Saturday, "The scene of that loch 'in full bearing' on a clear winter day, with its busy and stirring multitude of sliders, skaters, and curlers, the snowy hills around glistening in the sun, the ring of the ice, the shouts of the careering youth, the rattle of the curling-stones, and the shouts of the players, once heard and seen, would never be forgotten."

It is only eighteen miles to Bathgate from Edinburgh but to Simpson at that time the journey was too long to be made often. Communication with his family was thin—a letter cost 6½d. A travelling tanner sometimes acted as messenger and in the spring of Simpson's first year as a medical student, he brought an unexpected note from the old baker.

My dear Son,
I am glad to hear by John Pearson that you are well. . . . Be so good as to write to me what money you will take to bring you out. James, I am now turning old, and wearing awa like snow among the thaw. I have had a weary winter, but will be glad to see you at Bathgate.
I am yours in heart,
David Simpson.

Simpson spent the summer holidays in Bathgate. His interests now separated him from school friends, and he spent a good deal of the time completely alone wandering about on the low hills and farmland of West Lothian. His exercise books contained lists of birds, interrupted with random comments and queries such as: "Do male woodcock arrive before the female?" There are drawings of dissected birds with careful reference to their air cells—he attempted to measure the quantity of air, and compare it to barometric readings that he had compiled. Migration intrigued him and there is a list of rare visitors. "Is there a law governing stragglers as well as regular vistors to this country at particular seasons?" he wondered. His notes differ from other boy naturalists in their comprehensiveness, their capacity to see an idea through; to itemise *every* bird. Note-books full of geology and botany are equally systematic, with comments criticising his professors' accuracy.

During the holidays Simpson also helped the local G.P., the same Dr Dawson who had failed to arrive in time for his own birth. Simpson took over his dispensing, relabelled the bottles and tried to bring the country doctor up to date. The young student impressed Dawson's patients and was remembered by the village weavers and farm workers. One referred to him seventy years later as "a pleasant tempered, laughingly inclined lad . . . with enough pepper in him to season his sweetness into wholesomeness".

Simpson returned to the capital and had started his final year as a medical student when his father became il. He left Edinburgh at once, and for three weeks looked after the bedridden old man until the end. His death affected the youngest son deeply, the Simpson announced dogmatically that he would not go back and sit the final exams. The elder brothers and his sister Mary persuaded him eventually and pushed him off in the coach. Of course he passed the exams, and became a Member of the Royal College of Surgeons, Edinburgh at the age of eighteen. Too young, however, to complete the process and at once take his diploma and become an M.D. Simpson returned to his brother Sandy's house in Bathgate and wondered what to do next in order to mark time until he was twenty-one. Having enjoyed his time with Dr Dawson, he decided to be a country G.P., and applied for a vacancy at Inverkip, a little village on the Clyde. He went for an interview and was turned down. As he admitted later, "I felt a deeper amount of chagrin and disappointment than I have ever experienced since that date.

If chosen I would probably have been working there as a village doctor still."

Another brother, John, had maintained contact with a relation who had moved to Liverpool in order to increase his interests in shipping, and Simpson urged John to try to land him a job. John wrote and described the situation:

Mr Walter Grindlay,
    I understand from my brother at Grangemouth, that he had mentioned to you some time ago, that our youngest brother, James, had studied Medicine, and wished to get to be surgeon of a ship going out a voyage of twelve or fifteen months. He has been five years studying at the College of Edinburgh, and passed surgeon in April last. His ultimate intention at present is to take a degree as physician, and practise somewhere in Scotland or England; but he cannot obtain that till he is twenty-one, and he is only nineteen this month. As to his medical proficiency I am no judge, but a friend of mine, Mr Dawson, surgeon here, speaks favourably of him, and I know he is a good scholar, steady, upright, and attentive, and I think would be a good surgeon of a ship. He will require to attend the College another session before taking a degree, and his great anxiety at present is to procure a situation which will yield him a little, and where he can at same time see some practice. He is the youngest of us all, and a favourite, and we would be averse to his going in a ship designed for any unhealthy shore, but if you thought your extensive influence could procure him the situation of surgeon in an East Indiaman, or any ship sailing somewhere in that quarter for twelve or fifteen months, I would take it most particularly kind, and hope you will keep him in view should you hear of any suitable situation.

Mr Grindlay did find a ship post, but not until 1832. It was on the *Betsy*, under a Captain Petrie. By this time Simpson was lecturing in pathology and had to send his brother David to Leith "to advise Mr Petrie not to keep the situation vacant on my account". Petrie, however, does crop up again in the family story, and Mr Grindlay too.

David, the third son, had set up a baker's shop in Stockbridge, and James returned to Edinburgh to live with him and assist a Dr Gardiner. Simpson was glad of the holiday experience with Dr Dawson but he quickly realised the gaps in his knowledge: he discovered that he knew nothing of domiciliary midwifery and hastily began to attend extra-mural lectures on the subject. His aim now was to prepare for his M.D. degree and he presented himself in 1832. The first part of this exam was an involved interrogation in Latin, on medicine and surgery and then "Two Aphorisms of Hippocrates to explain and illustrate in writing". The second part was the presentation of a thesis. This had to be read by a leading member of the Faculty of Medicine, and then publicly defended by the candidate—all again in Latin (the practice was abolished a year later). Simpson's thesis was on inflammation—"*De Causa Mortis in Quileusdam Inflammationibus Proxima*"—and was allotted to the Professor of Pathology, Dr John Thomson.

Thomson was so impressed with this thesis and the author's ability in its defence that he immediately pushed through the swarm of students and, finding Simpson, offered him the coveted job as assistant.

At the end of the day Simpson had his M.D. degree, a very welcome job, and also a salary of £50 a year.

He wrote later, "Dr Thomson to whom I was then personally unknown, but to whose advice and guidance I subsequently owed a boundless debt of gratitude happened accidentally to have allotted to him my graduation thesis. He approved of it, engaged me as his assistant, and hence in brief I came to settle down a citizen of Edinburgh and fight amongst you a hard and uphill battle of life for bread and name and fame . . ." In a subsequent letter to the Lord Provost, when applying for the Chair of Medicine, Simpson was to write, "It was at Dr Thomson's urgent suggestion and advice I first turned my attention more especially to the study of Midwifery, with a view to becoming a teacher in this department." With this in mind, and a definite object in view, Simpson repeated the series of lectures by Hamilton, the Professor of Midwifery, during the winter of 1833 and '34. Why Thomson urged him to turn to midwifery we cannot quite make out. Hamilton's was the only Chair without a definite successor, and the Professor was getting old. Thomson was called scathingly by

Knox the anatomist "the old Chairmaker" as he had occupied several, and applied for more, but perhaps he knew that Simpson had the qualities for occupying some Chair, and it didn't quite matter which. Thomson felt confident that the young man would succeed in whatever sphere he happened to choose.

Professor Hamilton had very definite ideas, and his lectures were dogmatic. He was a fat little man, and used a sedan-chair, the last to be seen in the streets of Edinburgh. He wore a chestnut brown wig that did not fit, and walked with a quick noiseless step, peering down at his toes with his short-sighted eyes. He was always ready for a fight, and immediately reacted to any differences of opinion in his practice or print. He could not bear criticism, and   with a sharp tongue. His patients, however, adored him, and his practice was extensive in spite of his brisk manner and quarrelsome voice. His students also liked him, and he was popular as an examiner, provided the candidate followed the Hamilton line of thought. A contempory, Professor Robert Christison, writes,

I remember especially one occasion when he had in hand an Irish candidate who had got his midwifery in Dublin, where the teachers were, in Hamilton's opinion, heterodox throughout, and were the frequent objects of his professorial lash. The unlucky victim ran counter to the Hamiltonian creed in all his answers, and was too stolid to yield one inch to his examiner's argumentative interrogations. I accounted him a doomed man. But when Hamilton and I came to consult together he said 'Did you hear him? Did you ever hear such ignorance? I know he answers correctly as he has been taught in Dublin by a set of idiots. How can I punish him for their fault? I must let him pass. But as for trusting him with the delivery of a woman, I would not trust him to deliver a cat!'

It did not take Hamilton long to notice a particularly intent student in his extra mural class, older than the rest and working as the assistant of the Professor of Pathology. Strangely enough, Simpson never questioned Hamilton's authoritiative word, or entered into an argument, and professor and student became unexpected friends, embarking on a relationship that must have influenced Simpson in his ultimate decision to turn to obstetrics.

CHAPTER IV

Midwifery

IN 1870 A CONTEMPORARY of Simpson wrote, "Simpson adopted obstetrics when it was the lowest and most ignoble of our medical arts: he has left it a science numbering amongst its Professors many of the most distinguished of our modern physicians." To put the subject in perspective we must consider the background of childbirth through the ages, for the accoucheur of the nineteenth century had not come so very far in his art since the dawn of man.

In the most primitive communities, a woman remained alone when giving birth. Her menfolk would welcome the child, but be quite indifferent to the process of bringing him into the world. Later, and this represents a great cultural advance, the man remained with her and helped. Then came the phase of development when the man was not actively involved in the delivery but had a symbolic role to perform. Male Waiana Indians in the rain forest of Surinam still take to their hammocks and groan loudly in assumed pain. Marco Polo reported the curious custom of "Couvade" among the people of Chinese Turkestan 600 years ago: he described how the woman got up and went about her work immediately after delivery while the husband was put to bed with the child for forty days. Forms of this custom have been described from all over the world: Corsica, Ireland, Central Europe, as well as among the Bantu.

In a later cultural development, the husband was completely excluded and parturition regarded as an exclusively female concern, something to be kept from the profane male eye. Women of the family then gave way to outsiders with experience. Formal payment of these "wise women" was a later development, with arrangements made well beforehand for their attendance. These first midwives observed the process of birth repeatedly, and the simple and obvious things were done to help the woman in labour. Normal births proceeded normally. Abnormal births were attributed to evil spirits and to cope with this the witch-doctor, or later, the priest, would be reluctantly called in. He would try to coax the child out from its confined quarters and chase away the demons that were obstructing its path. The words and rites used differed slightly in each country and varied from age to age, but the gist was the same. The Victorian obstetrician had not much more idea as to why the child was lying the wrong way up than the witch-doctor. The actual process or birth had not changed during the ages; and the problems today are exactly the same.

Formal medicine is said to have begun with Hippocrates. By his time the midwife was a well-established figure. Under the law of Athens, it was essential that this woman be a mother, but past the age of childbearing herself. There were plenty of goddesses around to help her, Artemis, Hera and the authoritative Eileithyia who would increase the pains of labour as a punishment for any want of chastity on the part of the patient. It was considered by the people that the ability to choose the appropriate goddess was as important in the attributes of a midwife as her kindness and gentleness to the woman in labour.

The problems of Hippocrates were those of Professor Hamilton in Edinburgh in 1834. Puerperal fever killed off many of both doctors' patients after a normal delivery of a healthy child, and both treated it with purges and leeches, pessaries and cupping. Prolapsed uteri and sterility were complaints familiar to both. Hippocrates tested for sterility as follows: "Having wrapped [the patient] in blankets, fumigate below with oil of roses and if it appears that the scent passes through the body to the nostrils and mouth, know that of herself she is not unfruitful." Hamilton had not much more to offer his patients, but knew enough to consider oil of roses useless. The Grecian students learned to dilate the cervix and to use sounds to open up the womb, so as to gain access for fumigating and washing out the cavity using catheters of silver with various medicaments.

Grecian doctors were only summoned by the midwife as a last resort. When he arrived, the doctor would produce a few tricks which relieved the mother, but seldom the child. He could, for instance, turn the unborn child and would insert a finger into its mouth to help flex the head and provide traction for its delivery. The child by this time would probably be dead but hooked instruments were at hand to gouge it out if all else failed.

A book of instructions for midwives, *De Morbis Mulierum*, was written by Soranus, who practised in Rome in the second century A.D. According to Soranus, midwives should be well manicured, and also discreet for they were often trusted with family secrets. Two chapters were devoted to the special qualities that a midwife should possess, and there was a further comprehensive chapter on anatomy. Soranus upset many theories, particularly that the uterus had "nipple like growths, broad at the base and narrowing at the top, devised by Nature for the sake of teaching the embryo to practise beforehand how to suck at the nipples of the breast". The advice to the midwives was clear cut and his own treatments seem full of common sense. He does not approve of some remarkable older methods and does away with "giving the patient cold barley water to drink after suspending her head downwards on a ladder for a day and night to cure an inverted uterus. The cold drink causes flatulence and the prolonged suspension is uncomfortable." Soranus has a long dissertation on abortion in his book. Methods are reviewed and public opinion considered. "There is a disagreement; for some reject destructive practices, calling to witness Hippocrates, who says 'I will give nothing whatever destructive, deeming it the special province of medicine to guard and preserve what Nature generates'". Another author maintained the same view, but made an important distinction: "The fruit of conception is not to be destroyed at will because of adultery or of care for beauty, but it is to be destroyed to avert danger appertaining to birth." Hamilton, centuries later, quoted these words to his students, and Simpson copied them down in his notebook, with a query at the side.

Soranus's teaching of rational midwifery based on knowledge instead of superstition influenced the treatment of pregnant women throughout the civilised world. He discouraged the use of remedies for speeding up the arrival of the reluctant infant and was a great opponent of brute force.

The arrival of Christianity had a sad effect on the progress of midwifery. Faith healers became more important than doctors, and it was considered impious to dissect the human body. Sickness and disease were the punishments meted out by the Heavenly Father to sinful man and his even more wicked woman. It was a priest now who was called to attend a birth. The priest's duty was to baptise the child before it died. He had no concern for the mother, no interest in her suffering or the preservation of her life. It was thought more important that the midwife knew the words and form of baptism, than that she had any idea of basic anatomy and physiology. Baptism was the only way to salvation, and, ironically, legislation of midwives came into practice, not as a proof of their capabilities in the birth chamber, but as a verification that they knew how to christen the baby. The Continent at this time was far ahead of Britain in educating its midwives; for some reason it was less prudish, and there was not the same fear there of men learning intimate details of female affairs. If a handbook of midwifery should happen to fall into masculine hands the British priests felt that the men would be moved to "abhor and loathe the company of women".

It was not until the reign of Henry VIII that the first printed midwifery book appeared in English: *The Byrth of Mankynde*. The first edition was dedicated to "the most gracious Lady Quene Katheryne", and was written in Latin. Subsequent issues were in English, so that "the simplest Mydwyfe which can reade may both understand for her better instruction and also other women that have need for her helpe". The author is said to be Dr Thomas Raynalde, but much of the book is a translation and anthology of other people's methods. It reviewed the practices of the ancient Greeks; and Soranus, after 1,400 years, was in vogue once more. *The Byrth of Mankynd* approved of the "birth stool", a contraption more often used in France and Germany than Britain. The woman sat on the low horseshoe shaped seat, her back supported by an inclined rest, well padded with clothes.

The midwife her selfe shall sit before the labouring woman and shall diligently observe and wait, how much and after what means the child stireth itself. Also shall, with hands anoynted with the oyle of almonds or the oyle of those white lillies, rule and direct everything as shall seme best. Also the midwife must instruct and comfort the party not only refreshing her with good meat and drink, but also with sweet words giving her hope of a good speedie deliverance, encouraging and enstomacking her to patience and tolerance, bidding her to hold in her breath as much as she may, also stroking gently with her hands her belly about the navel for that helpeth to depress the birth duoneward.

Grecian teaching was also reviewed by the French Ambroise Paré, who re-introduced turning a baby within the uterus and extracting it feet first. This operation had been completely neglected for centuries, the woman and baby being left to die with nothing done to help, or subjected to mutilating operations that completely destroyed the child. Simpson referred enthusiastically and uncritically to Paré's work in his own lectures and often quoted directly from Paré's book. Simpson's copy, in vernacular French, was well thumbed, with numerous pencil jottings in the margin. On one page is a large exclamation mark beside Paré's account of a girl called Germaine Marie who fell while chasing some pigs. To her horror she had suddenly become male!

Ambroise Paré was a Huguenot. Catholic France was in arms against this sect of the church, and this persecution came to a head when Catherine de Medici and her family of Guises instigated the Massacre of St Bartholomew's Eve. In the weeks that followed more than 50,000 Protestants were slaughtered but a few did manage to escape and fled to the channel ports and across to the friendly shores of England. The Jervais were one family, and they continued their journey North to West Lothian as we have seen. The Chamberlens were another and they settled in London.

William Chamberlen had five children, two called Peter, who both became Barber Surgeons. The London Privy Council of Physicians disapproved of them strongly, jealous of their popularity with the Court and their influence with King James I. The Chamberlens could not become Fellows of the College as neither had been to Oxford or Cambridge, but the College was not yet "Royal" and the Chamberlens had the ear of royalty. The College retaliated by turning down the brothers' suggestions of instruction for midwives and by clapping one of them in Newgate. He was later released on the instruction of the Archbishop of Canterbury, a rare occasion on which ecclesiastic authority actually forwarded the course of midwifery.

The third generation of Chamberlens still had trouble with the College, and Peter Chamberlen III was "gravely admonished" by the President to "change his mode of dress and no longer follow the frivolous fashion of the youth at Court". He would not be made a member "until he conform to the custom of the College and adopt the decent and sombre dress of its members". This son stepped into the family shoes at Court, and tended to the Queen during various difficult confinements eventually delivering the future Charles II. He also took up the family cause demanding the education and the licensing of midwives, which brought even more criticism and accusation about his head. He published a public reply to these critics, "A crie of women and children echoed forth in the compassion of Peter Chamberlen." In this he blames the physicians and the Church for the ignorance of the midwives. "It is too greivous to think what a deluge of blood lies on their graves or conscience since these 30 years that my father attempted this charitie and 13 since I, in his example reviewed it." If Peter Chamberlen had had his way and been allowed to establish a school for midwives and been responsible for their licence, would he have told them the secret of why his family's methods of delivery were so successful?

Women of standing in the country all wanted to be delivered by the Peter Chamberlens. They had some method of shortening the agony of childbirth, but no one knew what it was. The Chamberlens went to much trouble to make sure that no one would! They would arrive for a confinement in a special carriage, along with a huge wooden box carved in gilt. Two people were needed to carry it, and its weight was supposed to be due to some massive complicated machine. The patient was then blind-folded, and the midwife locked out of the room. Relatives would glue their ear to the door and listen, petrified, to ringing bells and slapping of wooden sticks, sounds intended to disguise the clink of one metal blade on another. The Chamberlen's secret weapon was a pair of obstetrical forceps. With this scissor-like instrument they could carefully and safely pull on the head of the unborn child and hasten its delivery when the mother's efforts were not strong enough to push it out in time.

Peter Chamberlen III died in 1683, and his widow hid his box in the attic of his home, Woodham Mortimer Hall. There it remained undiscovered until 1813. Meanwhile three sons out of fourteen Chamberlen children became successful obstetricians with high class practices. Most influential was Hugh, who nearly let the family down by offering to sell out to the great French obstetrician, Francois Mauriceau. Mauriceau, however, refused to buy after Hugh and his miraculous instrument failed the test of delivering a dwarf with a twisted pelvis. She and her baby died after Hugh had delved under the bedclothes for three hours.

Five years after Hugh's death, however, the secret had leaked out, and a book appeared by Edmund Chapman in 1733 with engravings and a description of the Chamberlen forceps. From then on every obstetrician attempted to perpetuate his name by "inventing" a new modification. When the original Chamberlen instruments finally came to light, however, their design and material were agreed to be infinitely superior to any others. Many obstetricians obviously had thought along the same lines and, as is so often the case in medicine, an original thought burst through in several places at the same time.

Chapman's book opened a century that exposed many other secrets as well. A William Smellie practised as a doctor in Lanark, the birthplace of a surprising number of eminent medical men. He used various forceps in his daily work but complained that the midwives only called him in as a last resort. He was dissatisfied, too, with the French instruments that he was using, and apparently decided to go south and ask Chapman's advice; but London he found was a disappointing place "where nothing was to be learnt". This led him to teaching himself, and he was soon charging three guineas for a complete course in midwifery, with the students also paying 6/- to a general fund for the support of the slumwomen on whom they practised their skills. Smellie was inundated with patients, only too ready to be teaching subjects in return for the expert and kindly ministrations that they received from Smellie and his students. The instruments developed by William Smellie were used without modification up to recent days, and his method of practice combined with personal teaching was taken up by Professor Hamilton for use in the Edinburgh School. Smellie thought that it required much more skill to avoid, than to perform, obstetric operations, an idea much

quoted by Simpson at a later date. Smellie had his forceps made
in wood so that the patient would not hear the ominous clink of
metal or feel the icy steel of the blades. He would draw them
out of his pocket secretly under the bedclothes. It was considered that only men could handle instruments, and this had
gained them access to the lying-in chamber at last, but still
the prudery and prejudice remained, and only the most
brazen female would have let a man glimpse the process of
delivery. In Britain, and apparently even more so in America,
female modesty rigidly limited obstetrical investigation to
observation of the face and feeling the pylse, and palpations
only carried out strictly under the blanket.

In 1751 the obstetrician was still being instructed to sit
with a sheet or clothes before him, having his hands under the
cloth well greased with oil, Pomatum or Hogs hard without
uncovering any part of the patient, keeping out the external
air as much as possible". The forceps handle had to be large
to guide the poor doctor who was not allowed to see what he
was doing, and his sense of touch accurate enough to get him
over this difficulty.

One reason for the breadth of William Smellie's influence
was that his writings were edited by his best friend Tobias
Smollett. The novelist is said to have written Smellie's last textbook and certainly the literary style and readability of these
volumes are outstanding. Like the writings of Simpson, they
can be read by a layman with great interest and pleasure and
no unnecessary medical jargon is used to overcome any literary
deficiencies.

The teaching of midwifery in the 1800s was also influenced
by the work of a pupil of Smellie, another Lanarkshire lad,
William Hunter. He too followed the road to London, then a
tour of the Continent that included a stay in Holland. Here he
learned a method of preserving anatomical specimens, so
successful that his dissections are intact to this day, as a visit to
Glasgow Royal Infirmary's Pathology Department can testify.
Returning to London, Hunter began lecturing on anatomy.
Anatomists everywhere were now studying minute as well as
gross anatomy, and with his careful preparations and ability to
speak well he drew large classes. He was particularly interested
in the physiology of the placenta and uterus, and he began to

practise obstetrics, holding an appointment at one of the first
Lying-in Hospitals in London. It provided care for the married.
The unmarried were excluded from all hospitals except one
which came under the patronage of Queen Charlotte, which in
1791 allowed "poor pregnant women married as well as unmarried" inside its doors. The late eighteenth century was a
time of hospital developments throughout the country, and
1767 saw another opened in London "for the wives of poor men
and single women such as are deserted and in deep distress, to
save them from despair, and the lamentable crimes of suicide
and child murder". William Hunter was very interested in the
establishment of hospitals, for he was determined to promote
the acceptance of male midwives. Obstetricians were still not
eligible for election to the Fellowship of the College of Physicians and they were unpopular with their medical colleges.
Hunter wrote, "Physic is in a strange ferment here. The
practitioners of midwifery have been violently attacked . . . and
in that scuffle I have had a blow too. The reason is, we get
money, our antagonists none." The onslaught on male midwives came from the doctors and from the female midwives who
felt they were losing trade. However, the pregnant Queen Anne
and the ladies of the Court liked to know that a man was at hand
with his bag of tools, and Hunter's Scots tongue and ready
charm apparently made him extremely popular with the artisto-
cratic ladies of the West End. He was kindly and sympathetic,
and had that quality of inspiring confidence which makes the
difference between a competent and an outstanding obstetrician to this day.

Nothing furthers a personal cause more than treating the
wives of influential men, and Hunter had Lady Pitt as a patient,
as well as the Queen who, fortunately for him, had fifteen
children.

Literary London was fascinated by Hunter's preserved
specimens, and, attending his lectures, also fell for his charm.
His circle of friends included Oliver Goldsmith, Samuel
Johnson and Boswell. Joshua Reynolds also became a friend,
and the influence of moving in such cultural circles is shown in
the production of Hunter's textbooks of anatomy. Beautifully
illustrated with the finest engravings and magnificently bound,
they are works of art.

It is his anatomical research and study of the human embryo, not his way with the ladies, that has given Hunter his renown, although the money he extracted in medical fees paid for his celebrated museum; but it was his influence with the ladies of the Court that most furthered the cause of the "man midwife". He it is who is said to have had obstetrics accepted as a branch of the art and science of medicine, and the obstetrician accepted as a man of professional standing.

There had been a constant probing of ideas and problems during the eighteenth century, and with the invention of the microscope, the stage was ready for the major breakthroughs that happened during Simpson's time. Until now amputation of the breast had been practically the only operation carried out regularly to treat the particular ills of women; a Caesarian Section was only performed as a last resort to rescue a baby. For the most part the area between the breast and bladder was unexplored. Early in the nineteenth century, however, occurred an exciting event that was to herald the great surgical feats of the Victorian era.

Jane Crawford lived in Kentucky. She was forty-seven and thought that she was pregannt. Her labour pains began early in December 1809. They continued for a long time, but nothing relieved them. Two physicians saw her and, deciding she was heading for a very difficult delivery, sent for young Dr Ephraim McDowell who lived sixty miles away in the town of Danville. He had studied anatomy and surgery for two years in Edinburgh, then returned to Kentucky to become the most eminent surgeon west of the Alleghenies. He was also considered an able man midwife, so it was natural that he was called in to help Mrs Crawford. He arrived at her cabin in the hills on 13 December and quickly came to the conclusion that, instead of a baby, Mrs Crawford had a large tumour on her ovary. He told her blatantly that she would die, and soon, unless he tried to cut out the tumour together with the ovary, an operation which had never been done before.

"Having never seen so large a substance extracted nor heard of an attempt or success attending any operation such as this required, I gave the unhappy woman information of her dangerous situation," wrote McDowell in his diary. Brave Jane Crawford decided to put herself in the hands of the strikingly handsome, commanding young man, and agreed to go to his house in town and allow him to try to operate.

A few days later Mrs Crawford plucked up courage, rode her horse the sixty miles to town, and lay down on McDowell's wooden table. He was ready, having earnestly prayed for help. He later wrote the prayer down and gave an account of the operation.

Having placed her on a table of the ordinary height, on her back, and removed all her dressings which might in any way impede the operation, I made an incision about 3″ from the musculus rectus abdominis on the left side continuing the same 9″ in length. . . . extending into the cavity of the abdomen, the parieties of which were a good deal contused which we ascribed to the resting of the tumour on the horn of the saddle during her journey. The tumour then appeared full in view but was so large that we could not take it away entire . . . We took out 15 lbs of a dirty gelatinous looking substance after which we cut through the Fallopian tube and extracted the sac, which weighed 7 lbs and one half. As soon as the external opening was made, the intestines rushed out upon the table and so completely was the abdomen filled by the tumour that they could not be replaced during the operation which was terminated in about 25 minutes.

Jane Crawford afterwards told her grandson that she kept up her courage during the ordeal on the wooden table by repeating the book of Psalms. Her trust in them and the calm, masterly Dr McDowell was such that when he visited her five days later, he found her making her bed! Twenty-five days later still, she unhitched her horse and rode the sixty miles back into the hills, where she lived to be seventy-eight.

It was lucky for McDowell that his patient survived for they were both heading for the grave together that December afternoon. The men of Danville had collected in an angry crowd outside McDowell's house. They were awaiting the result of his surgical experiment. They looked upon it as an appalling piece of butchery and were ready to avenge the wrong inflicted on poor Mrs Crawford by the dreadful doctor. They prepared a gallows, and shouted through the windows, clamouring for his life. What effect this had on Mrs Crawford we shall never know. Another woman after undergoing a similar operation insisted that she had suffered much worse agony in her previous labours. However it seems incredible to our generation that any woman could submit voluntarily to such an ordeal and live to see it through.

Women were healthy in 1830, particularly in Scotland where the strong country stock was slow to die out. It was to be their children that developed the ills of the city life. Rickets and tuberculosis were not yet rife in the sunless slums. The new Lying-in Hospitals, though, were not turning out to be all that was expected. Babies were being born with more hope and less trauma, but mothers were dying. Infection set in a few days after the birth and usually proved fatal. It was noticed that if a midwife had one case, she soon had several, and that a crowded ward saw more infection than a woman in her own bed at home. Ideas of cleanliness were beginning to creep in, although people still considered baths as dangerous as fresh air.

Obstetricians from Hippocrates onwards had attempted to deal with the problem and Simpson was still looking for a solution in 1850, when he remarked that 3,000 mothers died in childbed every year in England and Wales.

CHAPTER V

The Young Doctor, 1832-1840

DESPITE HIS STRONG interest in midwifery, Simpson still devoted most of his time to pathology. His mind was not yet made up. Dr John Thomson was the first Professor of Pathology at Edinburgh University. This subject carried little weight in medical faculty circles. The chair had only been instituted in 1831, and was threatened with abolition ten years later, when Professor James Syme, the surgeon, said that "general pathology is not only unnecessary, but it is injurious because it teaches generalities, not specialities". Simpson, however, was influenced by his new chief immediately and he realised that the subject was a perfect background for every field of medicine. Dr Thomson was a man of great learning; cultured and cultivated but also very much of the world. He had previously held the Chairs of General Surgery and of Military Surgery, which led him to visit the army on the field after Waterloo. He was much influenced by the Continental schools and referred constantly to French techniques in his lectures. He denounced many of the current cures, particularly medical. Mercury was the indispensable remedy of the time, but Thomson considered it "pestilent and entirely pernicious". According to Professor Robert Christison, a central figure in University circles at the time, Thomson "professed an almost entire scepticism as regards almost all internal medicines, with the exception of rhubarb and soda". Thomson was also a philanthropist and, against much opposition, set up the New Town Dispensary in 1815, which was to give free medical and obstetrical advice and help to the poor in their own homes. Thomson's opponents felt that if people needed charity they must be made to come for it publicly and attend an institution. The Dispensary survived, however, and was flourishing by the time Simpson joined Dr Thomson. Although Professor of Pathology, Thomson was still very much involved in the Dispensary, and it was possibly he who drew Simpson's attention to the life of the poor, an interest in which he was to retain throughout his life.

Beyond Edinburgh Thomson was considered a leading authority in pathology. The new-fangled microscope was opening up the field of pathology and the time was just right for an enthusiastic young man to make good use of the new information, and to find flaws in many of the old theories. Simpson was given a free hand. As the chair was new there was no tradition of set lectures to be handed down, as was the case in surgery, where the professor, Munro, was said to be still reading the lectures of his great grandfather. The students reacted with a shower of peas when, year after year Munro III referred to the time when he was a student "in Leyden in 1719", yet he was never induced to change the dates! Dr Thomson, seeing the worth of his new assistant, apparently had faith in his learning and read Simpson's prepared lectures to his own class. Having delivered one of these to a room of students, he afterwards turned to Simpson. "I don't believe a word of it," he declared, and threw the papers on the table. Thomson later had to admit that even when he didn't agree with his theories, he was always impressed by his assistant's breadth of reading and attention to detail.

Simpson's notebook for February 1833 is a reflection of what filled his mind at this time. It is a hotchpotch of ideas; "Have in hand £13: Read Constantine (1289) for attack on Leprosy." Pages of prescriptions are mixed up with snippets of information.

In Parliament held at Compiègne they made some laws in marriage—allowed a divorce if V.D. contacted from husband . . .

Colic in West Indies because kept rum in bad barrels. . .

Fothergil speaks of lead in painted toys when applied to lips causing illness in children. Case in Worcester of 2 parents, 8 children died—lead in pipes.

Colic in Turnbridge when town water pipes of lead. Disappeared when changed to iron.

Constance's grandmother was natural daughter of Henry I of England.

Two pairs worsted socks.

Two pairs cotten.

Simpson was greedy for knowledge himself, and quick to see any gaps in other's. These he would then feel obliged to fill. Attending the various medical societies' meetings in Edinburgh, he was inevitably the first on his feet, questioning the speaker and suggesting he read the work of some often obscure writer, or filling in the details from the battery of references retained in his own very able memory. He did not care for physical research himself, but he made up for this by being completely up to date with other people's work and publications, those of American and Continental authorities, as well as of his contemporaries at home. Everyone soon knew Simpson and his name inevitably cropped up in the minutes of any society of that time.

The Royal Medical Society had the greatest authority in University circles. It dated from 1737, and was a platform for debate and the reading of original papers. These were dissected with great vigour and exuberance, and the Society's opinion was quoted in French and German medical circles as well as in London. Simpson was elected a Member in 1833, and also, in the same year, his old friend John Reid asked Edward Forbes to propose Simpson for membership of the Royal Physical Society. Forbes was the leader of the University literary set and was considered a brilliant young man. He was at the hub of the very active Society of Natural Historians and Simpson became closely associated with his doings. Forbes was slightly too intellectual for Simpson in some of his interests, and he did not become a member of Forbes's "Oineromathic Society, the brotherhood of the friends of truth". They were much in each other's company, however, canvassing for the Reform Bill and attending together the "Reform Jubilee" in Bruntsfield Links, close by the Meadows. Henry Cockburn describes the scene as "a beautiful and magnificent spectacle". At 10.00 a.m. the various trades and societies in and around the city assembled with banners, flags and music in Brunsfield Links. There were 15,000 of them, and another 40,000 looking on as the procession marched past.

They passed an address to his Majesty, the House of Commons and Earl Grey, and sang God Save the King, Rule Britania and Scots Wha Hae Wi' Wallace Bled.

This part of the ceremony was sublime and effective, the last song particularly which was joined in by thousands of voices all over the field with the earnestness and devotion of a sacrament. The anti Reformers had long predicted a riot their fond anticipations were disappointed.

Simpson also joined the band of young admirers who met to mourn Sir Walter Scott's death and consider a monument in his memory. One of the speakers was a young doctor, Douglas MacLagen.

Dr MacLagan was a lively young man, also involved with the New Town Dispensary. He was a great wit and story teller, and in later life his parties were considered the best in Edinburgh. He was very popular as an after-dinner speaker, usually turning on an impromptu verse. He and Robert Christison (both to become knights) were known as the "singing doctors" and performed at numerous gatherings of the Colleges of Physicians and of Surgeons, and the Harvein Society, as well as in aid of charity. They once made £70 for the benefit of a widow at a performance in St Cecilia's Hall. This caused some sensation at the time, as glee singing was considered somewhat infra dig for professional men.

Simpson had long wanted to visit the Continent, the source of so much original thought in medicine. His brother Sandy was prepared to finance a Continental tour, and in 1835, having finished his stint with Dr Thomson, he set off with his new friend, Douglas MacLagan.

Armed with introductions from Dr Thomson, the two young men made their way by carriage to London where they received excellent hospitality. It is lucky their hosts never read the comments they wrote home, such as this to the family at Bathgate: "How different is the drawling and simpering through a lazy French quadrille from the excitement of a 'guid' clithe reel or country dance."

To own a museum was considered a great social attribute, and there was much competition among medical men as to who had the largest collection. The Edinburgh doctors looked at dozens, toured the hospitals, listened to Pitt in the House of Commons and visited the zoo. Robert Christison, who visited London from Edinburgh at the same time, wrote

c

a full account of the medical scene, contrasting the two cities.

No other medical school offered the advantages of Edinburgh, he felt, where there was "ample materials for study, able superiors engaged in teaching, and ever on level with the times, museums and libraries freely open, professors and others to whom it is a labour of love to foster diligence and talent; a city abounding with all sorts of rational amusement; and good society easy of access." When Christison went to St Bartholomew's in London to further his experience he was very disappointed to find no one to teach him anything new. "Alas for St Bartholomew's! The pupil found no teacher, and more to teach others than for himself to learn." Ward rounds were made only once a week by the three physicians, and on one other day each saw a crowd of out-patients, that day being the only occasion on which out-patients could be admitted. Apart from this, the care of all the patients was in the hands of an apothecary, a little man called Wheeler "who was chiefly remarkable for his rare familiarity with the writings of Hippocrates". In any argument, "he floored Oxford, Canterbury and Edinburgh a little by quoting long passages in Greek". Christison remarks ruefully that he paid sixteen guineas to become a pupil, in return for which he "saw various intstances of deplorable results from the inadequate service in the Medical Department of the hospital . . . The worst part of the hospital discipline was the regulation, or rather non-regulation of the pathological dissections . . . and leave from the relatives of the disceased person was not, as in Edinburgh, a necessary condition." This meant that there was a race between the students and the relations, who wanted to grab the body first and carry it off intact. "Thus dissection was performed with indecent, sometimes dangerous haste on a body still warm and the limbs slack."

I remember one occasion [says Christison] watching the dissection of a man who had died suddenly one hour before. When cut open fluid blood gushed out. The Edinburgh visitors grabbed the arm of the dissecter to stop him going further and desperately tried to stop the blood coagulating on the table, like living blood. The London men roared with laughter, and eventually persuaded us the man was dead, but I never got reconciled to this summary off-hand procedure. . .

No wonder the Scottish graduates did well in the South, compared to the hundreds of doctors pouring into the ranks of the General Practitioners of England with a complete lack of knowledge of practical medicine.

Our other Edinburgh visitors, Simpson and MacLagan, talked to Lister who had long been the central figure in the Edinburgh surgical field and was now working in the North London Infirmary. They also attended an obstetrical lecture in Southwark Hospital, given by "one of the most popular lecturers in London". However they could not see the grounds for his reputation, the worst character of the lecture being "shocking indecency without qualifying wit . . . and the whole delivered with a flippant fluency" which, the visitors considered, was a very bad example to the young men.

However Simpson saw more in life than medicine.

19th April, 1835.

My Dear Sandy,

Do write me often. You cannot guess how I weary at times to hear from some of you. Before I received Mary's very kind letter last week, I was getting utterly uneasy, thinking something must be wrong that none of you had written. Dr M. and I met a very agreeable but small party of naturalists at dinner at Mr Speires this evening. We all adjourned to the Linnaean Society about 8 o'clock. The Duke of Somerset was in the Chair, and, honest man, fell sound asleep. . . . So sound indeed that he was with difficulty roused by the Secretary after the paper was finished and when it was necessary for him to speak a few words in order to adjourn the meeting. I shall leave London with the impression of having spent a most happy and instructive month of my life in it.

He adds in a P.S. that he "is amply supplied with money and needs no more".

Leaving London, the lush rich English scene impressed the Edinburgh men as they bowled along in the big coach towards the coast. They thought the suburbs of Southampton quite charming, and Southampton itself a very pretty town.

The whole scenery of the road was much more wooded than the generality of scenery in Scotland. The neatness and cleanliness of the English cottages is greatly superior to all that we have in Scotland,—the little patches of garden ground before, behind, and around them set them off amazingly. I wish the Scotch peasantry could, by some means or other, be excited to a little more love of cleanliness and horticulture. I did not see above two or three dirty windows, men, or women, along the whole line of road. The snow-white smockfrocks of the Hampshire peasantry do actually look well in my opinion.

Their passage across the Channel cost them one guinea, and they were immediately delighted with France. Simpson's letters were full of exuberance, and included snippets of information about French bread for his brother David and clothes for his sister Mary. Simpson loved the foreignness and Frenchness of the French: the fishermen with bulky petticoats and unwashed faces, the customs officers with cocked hats, moustaches and swords. He loved the women in their checked shawls kissing one another and chatting non-stop, using the muscles of their shoulders and mouths more expressively than words. He was struck with the liveliness of the scene as they travelled to Paris at seven miles per hour in the "Diligence Célérifère" pulled by five little horses. The postilion wore a broad-brimmed hat with a checked handkerchief round his neck and a dirty sleeveless jacket over green plush breeches. Luggage piled on top and the sixteen passengers sat inside or up in front beisde the *conducteur*.

Simpson and MacLagan darted from hospital to hospice taking note of everything, from the numerous gates and doors of the Palace with their French blue-coated sentries to guard the King and Swiss red-coats to guard the French, to the "coifs of some of the ladies that would have surprised you, at least they did surprise me. Many of them had no such thing as a bonnet on but a cap as high, or even higher than a sugar loaf made of muslin and lace and as white as driven snow."

The distinguished medical men in France gave the two young Edinburgh doctors a surprising welcome. British medicine, and midwifery in particular, was so poorly thought of on the

Continent that when the Duchess of Kent, Queen Victoria's mother, travelled from Amorbach, Bavaria, to England in 1819, she brought her own doctor with her. She was making her journey so that the child would be "British born", but not, however, "British delivered". Her doctor was Marianne Siebald whose presence was precaution against calling on such English practitioners as Sir Robert Croft who had been accused of "slaughtering Princess Charlotte through sheer incompetence". The lovely young princess had died of a haemorrhage after giving birth to a stillborn son. Not only was her adoring husband Prince Leopold desolate at this tragic event but the country was too. As the news seeped out of the Palace in November 1817 the British people realised that there was no one left able to inspire the nation: out of mad King George III's fifteen children there was no heir to the throne. The situation was saved by a hustle to the altar and the birth of Victoria at Marianne Siebald's hands. Dr Siebald had received her degree from Geissen University two years previously, after practising three years of midwifery, a fact that Simpson recalled at a later date, when he became involved with women doctors in Edinburgh.

The French doctors demonstrated their most interesting cases to the visitors, who noticed the disregard for the patient's feelings shown by their French colleagues as they discussed him across his bed. One professor made a point of considering the weather on the previous day which he felt had a direct bearing on the condition of his patients. He also went into great detail of the symptoms the patient did *not* have as well as those he did. The French students were apparently a very dirty, ill-dressed lot, and the surgeons not much better. One at the Hotel-Dieu operated in a dirty white apron, protecting a dirtier pair of trousers, a greasy threadbare coat and well-worn carpet shoes. He, M. Dupuytren had received Sir Robert Christison a few years before, and Simpson had an introduction from his Edinburgh friend.

The two doctors came home via Liége, which Simpson found "not so clean as Mons. Its environs wild and romantic. Besides it seemed full of good natured gash old wives and sonsy laughing faced, good looking, nay, some of them very good looking girls." They found time to climb spires and visit

Ruben's tomb and also admire a collection of drawings that had been used for William Hunter's great book. Simpson, a stickler for accuracy, pointed out that these drawings demonstrated various "discoveries" that had recently been claimed by French anatomists as their own! His active mind was stowing away a variety of facts to be shuffled, reassembled and reproduced at a later date.

Back in Britain, on their way north, the young men stopped at Liverpool where Simpson had a family connection. This was a cousin by the name of Grindlay—the same who had moved south to further his ship's chandler and trading business, and who had found Simpson the job as, doctor on the *Betsy* under Captain Petrie.

Simpson entered in his diary, "July 6th. At 7 I set off to drink tea and spend the evening with Mr Grindlay and his family . . . one of the Misses Grindlay has a resemblance to Mary. Much more like that of a sister than a second or third cousin."

Stimulated by his travels and full of enthusiasm, Simpson, returned home. The spotlight now began to fall on him as he stepped forward against a backdrop of the very able young men in Edinburgh in 1835. His first breakthrough was to be elected President of the influential Royal Medical Society, a much-coveted position among the up-and-coming post graduates.

Great weight was put on the inaugural dissertation. Simpson decided to blend his knowledge of pathology and his interest in midwifery, and to address the Society on "the Diseases of the Placenta". Here he commits himself to the subject for the first time.

For this he threw himself into amassing a fund of references and ferreting out obscure information from old books. He wrote to his French contacts, and a great number of people whom he did not know, in Germany, Belgium and in the provinces in the south of England.

He wrote to Sandy, as the day of the inauguration drew near, "It is 5 o'clock in the morning and I am confoundedly tired. I have been up all night correcting the last printed sheet of my paper. I was up all night on Monday—never in bed and have done with three or four hours sleep for several others." David, with whom he still lived, thankfully added in a P.S. that the paper was now finished and "happy we all are at it".

Work did not come easily to Simpson, but he was fortunate in having the necessary energy to overcome difficulties, and a discipline of mind that made up for any discrepancy between him and his medical contemporaries.

The paper on the placenta was a great success, not only in Edinburgh, where it was published in the Edinburgh Medical Journal in January 1836, but in France, Germany and Italy where it appeared in translation. It received a great deal of attention in the medical press and he was referred to as "the excellent Simpson" and his work accepted as a "very valuable compilation". According to the Italian, Dr Chelioni in Milan, it "filled up the void which medical science presented at this point", and Simpson from now on was considered the authority on the subject, an enviable position at the start of his career.

A visitor to the Royal Medical Society at this time wrote later of his experience:

On the evening referred to, the chair was occupied by a young man whose appearance was striking and peculiar. As we entered the room, his head was bent down, to enable him, in his elevated position, to converse with some one of the floor of the apartment and little was seen but a mass of long, tangled hair, partially concealing what appeared to be a head of very large size. He raised his head and his countenance at once impressed us. A poet has since described him at one of "leonine aspect". Not such do we remember him. A pale, large, rather flattish face, massive, brent brows, from under which shone eyes now piercing as it were to your inmost soul, now melting into almost feminine tenderness, a coarse-ish nose, with dilated nostrils, a finely-chiselled mouth, which seemed the most expressive feature of the face, and capable of being made at will the exponent of every passion and emotion. Who could describe that smile? When even the sun has tried it he has failed, and yet who can recall those features and not realise it as it played round the delicate lines of the upper lip, where firmness was strangely blended with other and apparently opposing qualities? Then his peculiar, rounded, soft body and limbs, as if he had retained the infantile form in adolescence, presented a *tout ensemble* which, even had we never seen it again, would have remained indelibly impressed on our memory. "You are in luck to-night," said our conductor, "Simpson is President."

Simpson was not as confident as one might suppose, and he confided to Sandy that the public speaking that he had to undertake as the President caused him a great deal of worry. Once he had to welcome the Principal of the University, a Presbyterian minister and had to refer to his own book, *Scots Worthies*, to find out how a minister behaved!

Now fast becoming evident was Simpson's capacity for kindling enthusiasm in others even when the subject in question was completely outside their interest and concern. There was much agitation in the spring of 1836 over the fact that the town's sewage was dumped, and had been for many years, into the marshy land to the north of the city. It was a hot May that year, and several enlightened citizens were beginning to take exception to the smell blowing back with the prevailing wind. In two days Simpson had talked 352 people into signing a petition for draining the marshes, all won over by his evidence of the insolubility of the marsh problem, although nothing had been done before.

Dr Thomson now became ill, and, after much arguing, the University Senate allowed Simpson to become Deputy Professor of Pathology. He had other intentions, though, and his interests were now committed.

As he wrote to Sandy in June of 36, "I have made up my mind to lecture on midwifery in Edinburgh. I am by no means as well prepared as I could wish, but I believe teaching the subject to others the best way to teach oneself."

In order to do this, Simpson had to buy a place in the extra-mural field. John Reid, his old friend, approached Simpson's brother John for a loan. Showing their usual kindness to the youngest son and confidence in this success, the family rallied and the brothers replied to John Reid, "Be as kind to him as possible and cheer him on. Sandy and I can easily raise £200 or £300 in the meantime. . . . Do not, if possible let James prospects be blasted, for I would rather that my own heart be broken than that he should be disappointed. I am sure I have told him again and again both verbally and in writing that he might consider mine as the joint stock purse of the family so long as it can be divided". John apologises for "not writing holograph"—an interesting point considering that his brother James was meanwhile publishing his works in the international journals and finding a place in the literature of the day.

Simpson now moved from his brother's shop, took rooms at Teviot Row and began to practise midwifery. "It is a most extensive subject and I sometimes become dispirited in thinking of it, but, if I do begin, I hope I will master it." As usual he immediately took steps to fill the gaps in his knowledge, and asked Professor Hamilton to find him a job in his Lying-in Hospital, an institution which Hamilton had founded, and supported now out of his own pocket. He used it to teach his students, saying proudly that, "a man saw as much midwifery [as a House Surgeon] during one year as he could expect to see in the usual routine private practice in the course of 20 years."

In having Dr Thomson and Professor Hamilton, his friends and his family behind him, Simpson demonstrates his great knack of mustering people to his cause. They all genuinely wanted to help, falling for his great smile and merry blue eyes. He is said to have had "no acquaintances, only friends". His buoyant enthusiasm warmed the heart, knocking aside apathy and involving everyone with whom he came in contact. Never indifferent to him, people either liked him or hated him.

The winter of 1836 saw the achievement of his immediate aims: he was lecturing in pathology, tending the difficult cases at the Lying-in Hospital and gradually building up his own practice from Teviot Row. "I am scarcely off my feet from morning to night, running after this and that." His patients were scattered over the Old and New Town; they were mostly poor, but he was optimistic. "I shall put a stout heart to a stey brae", he wrote to Sandy. "I do hope I may get into practice sufficient to keep me respectable." These were the days before the National Health. A doctor had no guaranteed salary to fall back on. He had to look for trade like the lawyer and the shoe-maker.

Despite his commitments, Simpson still had time to publish a paper to be included in a textbook of anatomy. It was on hermaphroditism, and referred among other illustrations to the sex of hens. To gather enough information, he had farmers throughout the Lothians and Fife scanning their poultry and

sending him off any of questionable sex. He sent them on to
Bathgate with a note that, "John perhaps will be so good as to
keep him, her, them or it and watch their habits till the plumage
falls". Sister Mary apparently suggested making Cock-a-Leekie
soup but was quickly discouraged by her young brother. Simpson was particularly drawn to the subject of Classical half men
and women, sons of Mercury and the goddess Venus. As with
all his other writings, this paper shows an extraordinary breadth
of source material, a passion for accurate classification, and a
capacity to unearth bizarre tit-bits of information. For instance,
who else knew of Maria Nonzia, a Corsican in 1695, who was
half man and yet married twice and lived for sixteen years with
her or his two husbands? Or who else would have uncovered
the fact that the deity Mithra was a hermaphrodite? The
bibliography at the end of the paper is formidable, including
Latin, Greek, French, Persian, Sanskrit, and American sources

Simpson snatched time to write between night calls and his
daily work. He tells Sandy, "Yesterday morning I was again
roused at 2 to a bad case, back by 4 and wrote till breakfast
time." He casually mentions in the same letter that he and his
friend John Reid had been elected Fellows of the Royal
College of Physicians of Edinburgh the week before and
continues with thanks for a pair of boots. The Edinburgh
cobbles in the Old Town had already gone through several
pairs, but he did not approve of the tackets his sister had
hammered in, as they were far too noisy, echoing up the closes
in the middle of the night.

With his tireless energy Simpson found time to dance, and
he and John Reid were considered very eligible by the mothers
of pretty young girls. The two were often to be seen at the
parties in the tall grey Georgian houses in the wide crescents
of the New Town. From references in letters we gather that
Simpson caused a flutter in many a heart. His own heart,
however, seems already committed in Liverpool, to Jessie
Grindlay who had so impressed him because she reminded him
of his much loved sister. His letters to her are strangely platonic
and businesslike, very different from the sentimental sonnets
that he was writing at the same time. She visited their common
relatives in Fife, which perhaps cemented their relationship, and
his letters became more frequent.

May 6th, 1836.

My dear Miss Grindlay,
Long looked and wished for comes at last—so be it.

He tells her that the local girl he has been seen in the carriage with "is a sweet and lovely girl, but not exactly the person who I think would make me happy, or at least happiest and since you left I have been presumptious enough to think for myself in these little items".

He next writes to her on his birthday, feeling sad at the way time is slipping past, wasted in sleeping, eating, amusement, ennui and idleness. "It was one of those days—those fitful days of gloom in which the past appeared to me as almost lost—the future as a labyrinth of vexations and disappointments and poverty and dependence." He asks her to write "and make me certain that you are my friend again", and sends her a book on geology and another on "apparitions". He also mentions that he has taken on a wager with Reid that he will be married before 15 August 1839.

He wrote again after another visit with John Reid to England in the autumn 1837. They returned by boat.

After we left Liverpool I sat musing on deck until sunset, and a beautiful and gorgeous sunset it was. By that time our vessel was dashing on most gallantly before a fresh but favourable breeze. Later Reid and I played at draughts till 10. We then came on deck to enjoy the night scene and such a night it was! I will not soon forget it. Our vessel was by that time joyfully and merrily dancing along the coast of Man with the wide and open sea for a ballroom . . . and the moon for a bright and laughing chandelier to it and an orchestra—but here my simile must really stop!
I feel perfectly lonely and out of the water since I returned.
Heigh ho,
J.Y.S.

He asks his sister Mary to offer Jessie a bed on her next visit north, and writes another letter on his twenty-seventh birthday.

My dear Miss Grindlay,

It is unfortunate that it is so as I do not happen to be in a pen pushing mood. I am not blue, no not at all but I have had a long day's work and I would not ask my eyelids to keep longer apart for any reason except you. Our dear cousinly self. . . .

It has been a year of wild downfalls and uprisings—of changing lights and shadows. Last winter was a strange blending of working and romping—of study and idleness—of pleasure and pathology, of lecturing and laughing, of agues and quadrilles, of insanity and coquetry. I had everything in excess except sleep and the paucity of it made room for the superfluity of everything else, good, bad and indifferent.

During the past year I have for once been outwitted by a lady and perhaps may be so again and again. . . . Next year shall I be married, think ye? and shall I have the pleasure of addressing you as sister? or not? If I knew it to be fact I think I would count out days of contentment, prosperity and happiness.

I was up at 3 o'clock finishing an essay for the next Edinburgh Medical Journal—I do not rise so early above once or twice a week, though I should do so. . . .

[Referring to gossip about a Miss Girdwood] she is, I confess a lovely young lady—but somehow or other I have come to think this summer that there is a great difference between a lovely sweetheart and a lovely wife between the beauty and ornament of the drawing-room, and that of one's domestic fireside and between a companion for the dance, and a companion for life.

As well as writing letters, Simpson was busy with his papers. He was well before his time in considering publications to be of the greatest importance. Medical journals in Dublin and London as well as Edinburgh constantly carried papers by him, translations appearing the following week in Milan or Paris. The next issue would print criticism and comment, so keeping his name to the fore. It was partly the influence of many literary friends and partly the need for ready cash that formed his habit of committing everything to paper.

The students attending the pathology course were most

enthusiastic, and the lectures obviously did not suffer from any luck of concentration on Simpson's part. It was customary for the students to present a Testimonial at the end of the year to the lecturer, and the one given to Simpson at the end of the 1837–'38 session is overflowing with admiration.

"We are anxious to express the high sense we entertain of the zeal, fidelity and success with which Dr J. Y. Simpson has discharged the duties of the Professorial Chair . . . as well as to express our admiration of his high talents and his uniform and kind affability, which while it exalted him in the eyes of all as a teacher, endeared him to each as a friend." The students championed the young Simpson, conscious as they were of the disapproval beginning to creep in from the established staff of the University. Edinburgh had always liked a show of character from its professors but they had to have reached a certain level of professional standing before they were allowed not to conform.

Simpson rather revelled in criticism from the establishment, and paid no respect to dignity. He also enjoyed success and was delighted with the enthusiasm of his class. His letters to Bathgate were particularly happy at this time, and those to Liverpool full of banter and teasing remarks. In one dated 12 April 1839 he tells Miss Grindlay that he has rented a house, with its own front door round the corner from his old lodgings, his brother lending him the money for the move.

He justified the new house and the luxury of a housekeeper from Dublin by the increase in his practice. His old landlady had been kind to him, but she tended to be rude to his patients and forgetful of messages. The new house was to cost £28, but then he had already made £90 in three months and could expect £300 before the end of the year from fees. Also he had the money from the lectures he gave twice daily.

These new lectures were on midwifery. The field had been made clear for him on account of the death of the extramural lecturer on the subject, a Dr McIntosh. Simpson taught the students the practical side of midwifery in Dr Thomson's dispensary for the poor, and also in the "Lock Hospital" which had been established by some worthy citizens for the care of destitute girls.

In spite of this increase in work, Simpson's name still appeared in the lists of social occasions and literary gatherings.

If there was anything going on in Edinburgh, he was there, somewhat untidy and usually late. His disarming smile and charm must have made up for any lack in social grace, and the Victorian families in Edinburgh enjoyed such apologies as:

> Dr. Simpson with great regret,
> Finds himself so much beset,
> With sickly dead and dying,
> As almost sets his eyes a 'crying,
> Hence ye of Number 23,
> Pray don't wait for him at tea.

that on one occasion he wrote on the back of his visiting card. The daughters of this family went with Simpson to the capping ceremony of the year's graduates, and one remembers that he pointed to Professor Hamilton and said, "Do you see that old gentleman? Well, that's my gown".

It is surprising that Simpson made so little attempt to foster the goodwill of the leading medical men in Edinburgh at the time. He never left anything unsaid. He was not the only one; feuds and controversy were the order of the day, surgeons bickering with physicians, anatomists publicly abusing the Chair of Midwifery, general practitioners taking umbrage at the merest slight on their behaviour and everyone prepared to take sides. Simpson though, made no effort to steer around trouble or let a critical remark lie. One acrimonious conversation in the rooms of the Royal College of Physicians was heading for a duel, until an onlooker hastily sent for the reliable John Reid to smooth down his friend and make the peace. Simpson was contrite and apologetic if he considered he had given offence, but if he felt strongly he spoke plainly, and then appeared surprised that feelings were hurt. He always meant well to start with, but his meddling was inclined to backfire. One of his more philanthropic acts that led to trouble had to do with the Lock Hospital, where he was one of the three visiting doctors. Venereal disease was rife at the time in Edinburgh, and the Lock Hospital was a charitable institution for the shelter and care of young girls in order to keep them off the streets. They however, were in return to conform to the rules of the Victorian middle class. Simpson fell foul of the managers of this institution by ignoring a rule that forbade the re-admittance of a girl if she had reverted to her old way of life on the streets, or had become involved with certain "establishments" in the city.

The girl in question was called Agnes Thomson. She had been in the Lock before, and, according to Simpson, "had always behaved with a degree of peace and decorum that was altogether exemplary and very much superior to that of the generality of our patients". She had made herself useful to him as a nurse. Cured of her venereal disease, Simpson had found her a job as a maid to a friend living in the country, and all was well for three months. But Agnes Thomson became lonely, returned to the city, and entered the house of Melbourne, which was of ill repute. She soon became reinfected and as she was then of no use, she was thrown out into the street. This brought her back to the Lock Hospital, but she was refused admission until Simpson appeared on the scene and was "moved by her pity and her wretchedness, and took her in" as he explained later.

The Reverend Lochlan McLean, the Superior, took exception to this disregard of his rule, and letters bristling with accusations and rude remarks were sent to and fro. A typical example runs:

Rev. Sir,
    The nature of your profession prevents me from answering your letter in the mode which it deserves.
    I am,
                            Your obedient servant,
                            James Y. Simpson, M.D.
Lock Hospital. 6th June 1839.

Simpson publicly accused the trustees of taking advantage of the girls in their care by forcing too much moral and religious instruction on them, and not enough medical help. He invited the reverend gentleman to meet him for a viva-voce explanation, but the mutual friend entrusted with the letter failed to deliver it, hoping presumably that the affair would blow over. He had not bargained with Simpson, however, who, "owing to the continued silence" of the Rev. McLean, now threw himself into a crusade on behalf of the inmates of the hospital. He involved the rest of the medical staff, wrote letters to the press, held a public protest meeting, and soon the institution was threatened with collapse.

At about this time Simpson accepted an invitation to visit Dublin, and we hear no more of the Lock Hospital. Then came a momentous turn of events: Professor Hamilton resigned. Immediately Simpson filed an application for the vacant chair and lodged it with the Lord Provost on 15 November 1849.

This chair was the first of Midwifery in the British Isles, established in 1726. The medical faculty at the time would have none of it. Its administration, therefore, fell under the auspices of the Town Council. There had been much argument between Senate and Council over the years, and in October 1825 the question arose as to what subjects were necessary for graduation. The Town Council maintained that midwifery be ruled essential, but the Senate refused what they considered to be an "outrageous proposal". The situation is described by Robert Christison in his autobiography. The Town Council was annoyed and marched in a body, complete with their robes, behind the sword and mace, to the University. They were received by the gowned professors, hastily marshalled in a line behind a long table. The Council commanded the Senate to obey their order, but the professors still refused to do so as they were told, or to take orders from such an ill-educated bunch of magistrates.

A lawsuit ensued but after much digging in old parchments, it appeared that the total authority of the Town Council over the University had never been repealed since the days of James VI. The indignant professors appealed to Sir Robert Peel and a Royal Commission was set up, which dealt with a great many things, but not the patronage of the chair of midwifery. "No good ever came to the University from the report of the Royal Commission", said Sir Robert Christison, who dismissed it as "utterly impractical and useless".

The brash Town Council were very proud of their authority over the intellectual professors, and exercised their rights by appointing the University secretary, janitor, librarian and porter, and even the class door keepers, although the professors were to be allowed the privilege of paying their wages. Most of the disputes between the Town Council and the Senate were solved eventually with the Universities Act of 1858, although some continue to make trouble to this day.

Never doing anything by halves, Simpson threw himself into the job of mustering ammunition to sway the Town Council to his favour and grant him the vacant chair. There were thirty-three members of the Council and it was considered fair game for each candidate to influence them in any way he could. The professors of the various faculties wielded enormous influence on the Town Council too. They had no actual vote, but the Council was inclined to accept their opinion. This led the professors to canvass openly for their favourite candidate and shower scorn and ridicule on the rest. On this occasion, they were unanimous. In their opinion, Simpson was not the man for the chair.

Their main objection was that Simpson was only twenty-eight (although this was not exceptional), with no social standing, background or esteem. On the other hand Simpson had done more for the science of his subject in a few years than they had in many, and in this lay his strength. His name was known to all who read their medical journals, on the Continent as well as at home. The work that he had put into his publications now reaped its reward and Simpson knew how to exploit it. But there were other difficulties, and Simpson was not too confident of the result as he confessed to his brother.

My dear Sandy,

I have all but given up hope of the Midwifery chair this time. Dr Lee or Kennedy of Dublin will probably gain it. I have been told by a member of the council that they have no objection by my youth and my celibacy and that if any person in Scotland gets it, I will. Notwithstanding these defects and you know I am superstitious—as much so as you yourself, and I dream always that I will yet be Professor despite of them, though not just now. I am in no way disappointed by their views. It will make me a Practitioner though not a Professor.

In great haste

Kindest love to all,

J. Y. Simpson.

Saturday morning.

The opinion of the day held that it would be quite indelicate to allow one's wife to consult an unmarried obstetrician. Realising this, Simpson immediately took steps to alter the situation to his advantage, and he wrote to Mr Grindlay asking for the hand of his daughter Jessie.

This letter reads like one of Simpson's scientific papers. It enumerates all the difficulties—he owes £200 to Sandy, wants to help his sister Mary emigrate to Tasmania, has borrowed money to furnish his house. However, as he says, he has a museum worth £200 or so and an excellent library. "All this I have won by my pen and my lancet, and these, as I have already told Jessie herself, as my only fortune. And now, could you trust her future happiness to me under such circumstances?" Mr Grindlay could and did. To the consternation of his friends, Simpson disappeared from Edinburgh at the height of the canvassing. The couple were married in Liverpool on 26 December 1839. They immediately returned by coach to the fray, and Simpson threw himself at the task of amassing as much weight as possible to wield against his opponents and impress the Town Council in his favour. The other candidates were meanwhile doing the same, but Simpson always tried to remain one jump ahead.

Edinburgh papers gave more and more space to the affairs of the University chair. Editorials appeared on the propriety of man midwives; the character of Professor Hamilton; the impossibility of ever finding another man of his stature to take his place, and, of course, they wrote about the candidates. Much weight was put on who, of influence in the town, was supporting who. Unfortunately for Simpson, the leading surgeon (now that Liston was in London), James Syme, was all for the Dublin Dr Evory Kennedy and said so openly in the press. The professors, including surprisingly Robert Christison of Materia Medica, who had obtained his first chair at twenty-five, announced that they considered it blatant presumption that one so inexperienced as Simpson should consider himself a serious competitor.

Simpson's friends tended to be young men, as irritating to the old school as Simpson was himself. Well aware of this, he turned his attention farther afield and with his new wife's help, wrote to everyone who could be of the slightest influence, asking for their confidence and a testimonial of this support. He drew their attention to his publications and the enthusiastic reception of his work in the pathology and midwifery fields.

Quoting liberally from the replies, Simpson drew up his curriculum vitae, which he printed and posted to all who he considered could influence the Town Council. The document begins with a clear cut synopsis of his jobs and experience, then come critical comments by his students on his lectures in pathology and midwifery. A formidable list of his publications follows, including translations and remarks which, it is pointed out, were written long before the present vacancy occurred, by eminent Continental authorities. After that there are references, beginning with those of twenty-seven professors or lecturers in midwifery, followed by the opinions of the most eminent accoucheurs in Great Britain and some of the most distinguished members of the medical profession in France, Belgium, Switzerland, Germany, Denmark and Holland. It is, as Simpson writes in his covering letter, a "Testimonial which requires no comment". Reading it, one wonders who else could possibly be more qualified for the chair. However, the establishment was not easily swayed, and the University and the Law were expected to be for Kennedy.

Just before the election Simpson wrote to his father-in-law.

I have no more time than to say how extremely thankful I feel for your last loan. This horrid canvass has almost completely emptied our purse and Jessie and I were beginning altogether to lose heart, when your kindness, your great kindness, has again restored it. The canvass stands thus— Dr Kennedy and I are about the only candidates (there are 33 votes and I have secured 15 of them. If I can manage to get 2 more which is extremely dubious yet—the chair is mine.

Jessie and I were up at 4 in the morning writing the last part of a catalogue of my museum. It is now nearly 12 at night and I must go to the High Street to look after the printers. I will slip in this as I pass in the post—but as the money office is shut at this late hour you will require to pay 2d. for it.

Excitement grew intense as three of the original five candidates dropped out and left the field clear for a straight fight between Simpson and Kennedy, who held the post of Master of the Rotunda, Dublin. Newspapers began to take sides, Whigs and Tories became involved. It was now noised abroad that Kennedy was a poor lecturer, while Simpson, as was well known, was particularly good. To squash this rumour, Syme and other of Kennedy's friends brought the Irishman to Edinburgh and he delivered a public talk in the Assembly Rooms. His audience however, was not impressed, and acid comments appeared in a surprisingly unexpurgated form in the public press. Kennedy had 200 specimens in his museum. Simpson hastily added to his, and published a new catalogue with slightly more. He wrote again to Mr Grindlay. "Having written and canvassed nearly 17 hours I felt so ill as to apply to my medical friends who sent me for a drive through the woods along the Forth to Dalmeny. If only you were here to see the bustle and turmoil connected with the closing weeks of the canvass."

The *Edinburgh Weekly Journal* of 29th January carried a big editorial beginning, "We have no rememberance of so keen a contest for a medical chair as exists at present." The excitement of citizens, professors and students grew intense as Tuesday, 4 February, Election Day, drew near. The supporters of Kennedy honestly believed that he was the better man—not as an obstetrician, that was beside the point, but as a person who would add dignity and distinction to the University. Simpson accused the professors of "having a dread that a poor baker's son should be made their equal" and perhaps he was right, although such feelings are not characteristic of Scotland. If he had not won over the University, Simpson had certainly captured the affection of the citizens of Edinburgh. He was a Scot—one of themselves. "A vernacular man", as Carlyle said of Knox, "Scotch every bit of him, Scotch to the marrow of his bones." He had no airs and graces and none of the academic disdain to which the ordinary man might take exception. He cared, and this was readily noticed, which explains his rapidly snowballing practice. He was as big an Empire builder as most ambitous men, but he could put this aside to respond honestly to the needs of another—disregarding the rules or system. That this warmth and concern, the approachability of a young man of twenty-eight, was so evident and widely commented on is unusual and worth remembering.

When the day arrived, every member of the Town Council was present—a very rare thing. Lord Provost Forrest himself proposed that Dr Evory Kennedy be appointed. Baillie Ramsay proposed Simpson. The public area of the Council Chamber was packed with students, those studying classics and arts as well as medicine. According to Christison, the entire Royal Medical Society was packed in, as well as a strong contingent of Irish. The Council retired. The result was awaited with bated breath.

At last the count was declared. Sixteen votes for Kennedy, seventeen for Simpson. Cheers resounded loud and long in the streets as well as in the quadrangle. Simpson's reaction is displayed in his brier letter to his in-laws.

My dear Mother,
    Jessie's honeymoon and mine is to begin tomorrow. I was elected Professor today by a MAJORITY OF ONE. Hurrah.
                    Your affectionate son,
                    J. Y. Simpson.

The only letter of congratulations among the hundreds that Simspon himself retained was from his sister Mary, now emigrating to Tasmania. "My dear dear and fortunate brother ... I never believed till now that excess of joy was worse to bear than excess of grief. I cannot describe how, but I certainly feel as I never did all my life."

Where the honeymoon was spent is not quite clear but not long after the election Simpson published an article referring to archaeological relics on the Isle of Man.

CHAPTER VI

The New Professor, 1840-1847

THE NEW PROFESSOR sat squarely in his chair, well aware of the discomfiture among the occupants of the others. It was not in Simpson's character to leave anything for time to heal, nor was he preapred to placate the frosty Senate by adopting the role of subdued new boy. But he was far too good-natured himself to harbour a grievance for long, and his mind was too active to dwell on past animosity. "Never nurse a grudge," he said once to a friend. "It's as uncomfortable as a cold hot water bottle."

The Professor of Materia Medica had been one of Simpsons antagonists in his fight for the chair. This was surprising, as Robert Christison and he had moved in the same set, shared friends, and both admired the fire and character of the other. Christison loved the hills, and the first friendly contact between these two men after Simpson obtained his chair seems to be the sharing of a carriage out to Liberton, two miles south of Edinburgh in the Spring of the year. Christison set off for a walk up into the Pentland hills, while Simpson trudged over a field to look for the site of an old hospital. He thought the name of the village a corruption of "Liper Town", indicating that a leper hospital must have existed somewhere near. He was becoming interested in the prevalence of this disease in the past in Europe and in Scotland in particular.

Sir Walter Scott's friend, David Laing, was also in the party, having come to show Simpson the "oily well of St Catherine's" at Liberton, which was alleged to have cured leprosy and was famous well into the seventeenth century. It was claimed in a "Memorial of the rare and wonderful things of Scotland" of 1612 to cure "all salt scabs and tumour that trouble the outward skin of man", and King James VI made a special journey in 1617 to see it, and ordered it to be protected with a brick wall, later pulled down by Oliver Cromwell.

No doubt as well as archaeology, David Laing talked of his new appointment as Librarian of the Signet Library, It was said of Simpson that he quoted from books that no one else knew had ever been written, and probably David Laing was the source of many of his more obscure references. Laing was said by Sir Walter Scott and also Carlyle, to be very free with his fund of antiquarian knowledge, and Simpson seems to have been particularly adept at extracting information from his companions. Laing also kept Simpson in touch with the literary world farther afield than Edinburgh, and, although never an intellectual himself, Simpson appeared to be at home in their company, and welcomed into their set.

Robert Christison was a prodigious writer too. In one year 1840 he edited the *Edinburgh Medical Journal*, produced a thesis on the kidney, a text book on poisons and also numerous papers on fever. He was considered the ultimate authority on Materia Medica, and was said to be the instigator of Medical Jurisprudence in the United Kingdom. He was constantly called by the Crown to give evidence in trials, the most famous being that of Madeleine Smith, the respectable Glasgow girl accused of poisoning her Italian lover. Oxalic acid was the favourite poison as most good Victorian households had it readily at hand. The maids polished the brass with it and used it to put the shine on the fashionable yellowed tops of their boots.

Christison's experiences in the courts were enough to intrigue anyone, let alone someone with a curiosity like Simpson's, and he often alluded to his friend's cases in his lectures to his class, There was, for instance, the case of the brothel keeper, a powerful woman and notorious fury, charged with murdering a law clerk in her house by stabbing him in the chest with the point of the carving knife. The body was examined at the Royal Infirmary, and a gash was found in the left ventricle of the heart. But Christison was an impartial observer at the time, and noticed that the knife, after cutting the cartilage of the 2nd left rib, had penetrated inwards and downwards. This fact proved to be of great consequence. The woman declared that the young clerk and his companions had become drunk, uproarious and rude, and that she had seized the knife in self defence; she had held it up in front of her, and the young man had stumbled towards her, on to the point. One of his friends, on the other hand, swore that he distinctly saw the woman hold it dagger-wise, raise her hand to her left ear and strike downwards. On Christison's evidence she was found guilty of murder, condemned and executed.

Christison must have drawn Simpson's attention to any interesting cases coming up in the courts, for jotted in his note-book of this time are references such as "Christison—High Court 11". Simpson's own appearances in court were usually connected with abortion or cases of illegitimacy and inheritance. This led him to endless research into the question of the length of pregnancy. He published a paper on the subject, which considered the gestation period of hens, sheep and cows as well as referring to such authorities as Artemis, who coped with the celestial labours of the Ancient Greeks. The cases Simpson refers to invariably seem to have a slightly bizarre addition to the point in question, such as the lady whose pregnancy lasted eleven months, but then

the previous January 4th a large steamer in which she was travelling to London, caught fire when 2 or 3 days out at sea and only a small number of the passengers and crew escaped. After making almost superhuman exertions to save herself and a young son 17 months old, whom she held in her arms, and after having her body severely bruised and contused, she was exposed for 17 hours in an open boat with little or no clothing, and sitting immersed several inches deep in water during the whole of that long and anxious period. Yet all that fearful mental excitement and bodily exertion to which she was subjected were accompanied by no tendency to miscarry. Could this mental agitation have led, in fact, to the unusual prolongation of her pregnancy?

Simpson's mind was perhaps dwelling on pregnancy because his own first child was born just then.

To Mrs Grindlay, October 16th, 1840.
My dear Mother,
    Jessie keeps *amazingly well*. She seems perfectly delighted af having got her work over. I wanted her to wait till the 3rd ot

November when the delivery of my introductory lecture would have been a more appropriate date for commencing. I wish I was delivered of it now.

Your soncy, rather sedate little granddaughter has done nothing but sleep and sip sugared water all day. Poor little "bodie" what else has she to do in this world yet?

Your affectionate son,
J. Y. Simpson.

Saturday 8 o'clock.

There are many indications that he loved this child, and seemed to shower on it, and indeed all his children, far more affection and exuberance than was typical of a Victorian father.

My daughter, oh my daughter [he wrote to his sister-in-law soon after the christening] I do love the little marmozette so. She said not a word on Monday—was asleep during the ceremony. Won't answer yet to Maggie. Cannot get my tongue round Margaret. Jessie makes a famous nurse.

I got [sister] Mary's picture up to grace the baptism. May God bless her I do think my little daughter's like her.

The hall was packed for Simpson's first lecture as Professor of Midwifery. A carriage had come from Bathgate bringing the local practitioner, Dr Dawson, and the schoolmaster, one brother and other friends to swell the ranks of the students.

Simpson was elated, and afterwards wrote to his sister-in-law,

Have intended to write for days and weeks past, but very busy and every moment is gold. Am delighted of course, with the class. Had to apply to the council for additional sittings and again for some days students standing for want of seats. For the first time in the history of the University, the Midwifery is the largest class within its walls. It is very satisfactory to beat in the race not only my *friends* of the Medical Faculty but all the 30 bald and grey headed professors. Dr Allison, who changed his hour to lecture at the same one with me, has a very small class. Don't he deserve it? He has broken his own head and missed mine!

Do you know, I sometimes fancy the students 'gane gyte' when they come crushing into the room to hear *me* lecture.

"The art of teaching is the art of sharing enthsuaism", has been said by a current Professor of Midwifery in Scotland, and Simpson obviously believed this maxim too. His lectures were concise, clear and direct. He would write some cryptic headings on a blackboard, then proceed methodically to explain. His only notes were jottings of references—Biblical texts or Ancient Greek. A letter at the time comments on his "fluent and chaste diction—the orderly clear and logical arrangement of his ideas and the warmth and fervour which he enabled to throw into his addresses, having a powerful influence in awakening interest in the subject itself and keeping alive attention to the instruction he was communicating".

The students copied down the lectures, and a prize was presented to the one with the fairest head. These prize-winning books have been retained in the library of the Royal College of Physicians of Edinburgh. They make most interesting reading. Few medical lectures of today could be attended by a layman with any interest, let alone comprehension, but Simpson's were packed with pertinent anecdote and vivid personal recollections. He gives the impression that his mind was seething with ideas which he hands out, feeling for solutions as he goes along.

The reader is also made ware of his kindliness and compassion—"make sure that the patient is not upset", "she will prefer to . . .", "she will be eased if you . . ." Flashes of insight into the social scene are given, as, for example, in Simpson's warning to his students to be sure of their diagnosis; otherwise, he tells them, they may be in trouble in the courts. Action for damages were readily taken out by the mistresses of maid-servants whose doctors thought their pains due to abortion and sent them off to the Lying-in Hospital, while in fact many turned out to be suffering from dysmenorrhoea. Any reflection on the morals of the Victorian household caused great indignation. Female feelings were always considered in Simpson's lectures, and the students were urged to draw the curtains and use gas light when examining a patient, in spite of the fact that daylight would have been much more efficient.

To prove the source of one story, Simpson read a passage in

Latin. One of his students scribbled a remark in the margin of his book. "This passage was read in sound and healthy Latin untained by Cockney accents." Apparently too many Scots were getting slovenly over their speech and "assailing our ears with the most disgusting and contemptible pronounciation. Humbling it truly is, that Scots physicians, known in former days for their beautiful reading of Latin, should ape the set of English snobs!"

Among Simpson's papers, jotted down in his hasty writing, is a scrap of paper for reference during one of these lectures. It reads:

Deaths during first year of life 1 in 4½
In Prussia 27 out of 100
France 21
Amsterdam 22
Sweden 22.

These were the days before statistics became common language, or Government White Papers readily available, and one can only guess at the amount of letter writing involved in procuring such information. Simpson was years before his time in using such facts and figures in forming medical conclusions.

"Know the technique by all means, but don't disregard the application," Simpson repeatedly rules "else you will resemble the learned Dr Hewell who read all the theory of skating but could not keep his balance on the ice, remarking as he fell down 'I am up in theory but down in practice'."

"We are getting far too sophisticated," was another of Simpson's principles. "Let's get back to normality . . . Drs Rigby and Ramsbottom rush and rupture the membranes before they take time to get their coats off. I prefer to wait."

Simpson advocated action when necessary, of course, and had a story to prove the point.

It happened that I received a note during one of my lectures, but I could not read it at the time, on account of its being so badly written (and there was a good reason, I afterwards discovered, as the attendant had written it with his left hand, the other being kept all the time stemming back the blood).

However, at the end of lecture I found a person waiting for me with great anxiety, asking me to go with him. We rushed down the High Street to the Canongate, and found the child stuck. The mother was dying, so I immediately cut up the os uteri on each side and soon got away the child. There was much haemorrhage, but by the use of the sponge plug the patient recovered—and this season she was delivered of twins.

Simpson enjoyed the contact with his students, far more so than that of his colleagues. Active partisanship on the part of the other professors does not seem to have upset Simpson at all; acts like that of Dr Allison who changed his lecture hour to clash with Simpson's class gave him welcome justification to slate the Senate, which he did with relish and at every opportunity. The ladies of the town loved this, and began to urge their general practitioners to send them to the young and outrageous professor for obstetrical advice. There was no room in the Simpson house in Dean Terrace for this increase in practice, and the area was not elegant enough for the more prosperous patients now knocking at his door. So Simpson decided to move up the hill towards the centre of the town. He also now needed a carriage. He asked Sandy to lend him the money, jusifying his extravagance by the saving of time and the need to support his rank among the wealthier doctors of the town. Mr Grindlay also offered to help, and Simpson accepted with alacrity. He was absolutely confident that he would soon be able to pay back his debts, plus an interest on the loans.

Money may have been a motive for the amount of work that Simpson undertook, but there can be no doubt of his enthusiasm. He still trudged up and down the tenement stairs to visit the scattered patients of his original practice and his wife wrote ruefully to her sister that he was "wont to spend his time with the poor and forget to collect the fees from the only patients with the money". She would have been furious to know that her husband had answered a begging letter and had lent £50 to a casual friend at this time "till his fees came in in a new practice in England".

However, despite his apparent disregard for money, Simpson repaid Sandy his first £100 in the September and wrote with conviction that he could "without inconvenience send another £100 in a month".

Papers continued to be written during the night, between calls, but even this was not enough. Dr Sharpey, the Professor of Anatomy in the University College of London wrote to Simpson, saying that the publisher of his medical works was in utter despair for his material; he advised Simpson to get on with the job in hand and not become so involved with petty arguments. "Write your paper", urged Dr Sharpey "and put for a motto 'Despectu Inimic-orum' as Frederick did when he built a palace in the middle of the war." It is significant that Sharpey was a friend of Professor Syme, and therefore unlikely to be sympathetic towards the pushy young obstetrician.

Simpson produced the manuscript, and also managed to complete a marathon paper on the incidence of leprosy in Great Britain, which he read to the Edinburgh Medical and Chirurgical Society. This subject satisfied his growing passion for archaeology; yet justified his time by being vaguely medical. The paper demonstrates his ability to extract material from every conceivable source, and shuffle it into readily readable order. It had 500 references to ancient manuscripts and books, all read and digested, and quoted numerous letters answering his queries from religious orders and country parsons throughout the Continent and Great Britain. He was particularly interested in the incidence of the disease in Scotland, and ferreted out the information that Robert the Bruce founded a hospital for Lepers on the bleak moor at Kingsacre near Ayr, and that the Lady of Lochow had erected one in the Gorbals of Glasgow, beside the Old Bridge across the River Clyde. The inmates had to carry clappers and walk only in the gutter side of the street and hold a cloth over their mouth. These hospitals were intended as places of seclusion, and not for any cure, although, according to Michael Scott, the Fife philosopher "it ought to be known that the blood of dogs and of infants 2 years old or under, when diffused through a bath of heated water, dispels the leprosy without a doubt". The inmates of the leper hospitals had to "live quitely and give no scandal by swearing, flirting or filthy speaking, and say their prayers 32 times a day". Those in the Edinburgh Hospital were given 4 Scotch shilling a week (about 4d sterling) and were obliged to beg at the hospital gate for any more, but most English hospitals were well endowed; founded to secure spiritual peace and pardon to the donor and his family, some were even rich enough to dispense free and unlimited beer to their inmates! The lepers of Sherborne for instance had a daily allowance of a loaf of bread and a gallon of ale each, with fresh salmon on the feast of St Cuthbert in Lent. Lepers in France, however had to watch out that they were not burnt alive. This not only cured the infection of the body, but also purified the soul of the afflicted.

The disease was rampant in the north long after it was eradicated in England. In 1740 two lepers died in Shetland, and the Session Book notes that the Parish paid for the tobacco. Was this, queried Simpson, used as a preventive or disinfective agent? In some districts of Scotland in the present day all the attendants at a funeral are regularly provided with tobacco and pipes at the expense of the relatives of the dead person maintaining the same tradition. Simpson's paper continues at great length with fascinating details of leprosy in Iceland and even Greenland, and of the disease breaking out in St Kilda in 1697. On this most westerly island of the Hebrides the peoples' "feet began to fail, their appetite decline, their face becoming too red, a hoarseness, and their hair falling out, with their beards growing thinner than ordinary". The disease did not even spare the Royal Family of Scotland, and in 665, the heir to the throne, Fiacre, was "so full of lipper that he was repute the maist horrible creature on earth" (Œuvres de Rabelais, 1835).

Simpson had even more information on the subject: who else knew that Henry III of England courted Margaret, Princess of Scotland, but that she preferred the brave Hubert de Burgh, the minister of the English king? No wonder, for Hubert alleged that Henry was "a squint eyed fool, a lewd man, a leper, deceitful, perjured, more faint hearted than a woman and utterly unfit for the company of any fair and noble lady". The great Robert the Bruce was also struck with the disease, which prevented him from leading his army into England in 1326. It also rendered him unable to attend the peaceful nuptial feast of his son at Berwick in 1328, and "he became aged and feeble and greatly changed with the sickness so that there was no way with him but death", although his mind was active and vigorous right up to the end. During the very last year of his life he ex-

perimented in ship building and navigation while in retirement at Cardross Castle, near the banks of the Clyde. Just
before his death he wrote the well known wish, charging his
favourite friend "Ye gentle Knighte of Douglas, I will that, as
soone as I am trespassed out of this world, ye take my harte out
of my body and embaume it, and present it to the Holy
Sepulchre at Jerusalem, saying my body can not come".

The paper was received with great admiration by the Archaeological Society, who urged Simpson to print it in full.

Simpson followed Dr Sharpey's advice to keep out of trouble
for a while, but was quite unable to stand aside when the Senate
decided to abolish the Chair of Pathology in 1842. He became
completely involved, championing it against all odds. His
leading opponents were, of course, Syme and Allison, who
had decided that the chair was quite unnecessary and should be
abolished on the retirement of Dr Thomson, who had instituted
it and occupied it since 1837.

The College Committee summoned the medical professors
to a conference to decide the issue, and they were invited to
submit their opinions in writing. Simpson immediately printed
his in the form of a booklet and offered it not only to the
Committee, but to the citizens of Edinburgh, the Houses of
Parliament and to the press, aunouncing publicly that "I have
the misfortune to differ in opinion from the great majority of
my colleagues". His argument was that the scientific teaching
of the causes and results of disease would be crowded out of the
medical curriculum by the teaching of the practice and remedy.
"Unless some most unexpected change takes place in the human
mind, then Medical Science must progress, swelling out to
require more chairs, not less."

The controversy was followed with interest by the town: and
no wonder, since the professors rushed into print on every possible occasion, outdoing each other in sarcasm and barbed wit:
"For merit of the discovery of the most original objection to the
Chair of Pathology my colleagues are indebted to the zeal of
Professor Syme . . . but the College Committee will pardon me
for not troubling them with any formal reply to such a ridiculous argument". Was Simpson's tongue in his cheek? His
trump card was a printed letter from James Clark, the Queen's
Physician, endorsing all that Simpson had said.

London, September 20th 1841

My dear Sir,

I am indeed astonished as well as grieved to find that there is a risk of the Chair of General Pathology in the University of Edinburgh being abolished . . .

. . . I regard it as a course absolutely necessary to complete a good medical education and it is extraordinary that the patrons of the University should endeavour to crush a branch of Medicine rising up everywhere else.

I shall indeed lament to see my Alma Mater, the Medical School that stood pre-eminent in Europe, make a retrograde step which must lower her character in the estimation of all Europe . . . I entreat you to use all your efforts to avert it and with sincere wishes for your success in so good a cause, believe me.

My dear Sir,
Very truly yours,
J. Clark.

Robert Christison, a friend of Syme, Allison and Simpson, seems to have been attacked by all three. His only printed comment questioned the accuracy of various allegations by Simpson concerning history of pathology. He commented shrewdly that, had he been an autocratic University Rector, he would "be disposed to apply the jocular recommendation of Lord Brougham to the Council of the University of London, that for the sake of peace between its walls, the professors should be forbidden to print anything short of an octavo of 300 pages".

Simpson's persistence wore down the Town Council once more, and the chair was retained. Simpson suggested that a Dr William Henderson should be appointed as a successor to Dr Thomson, little realising that this would involve him in his bitterest battle yet, although this time some of the establishment were actually to be on his side. This came about because Dr Henderson announced himself to be a homeopathist. The subject of homeopathy was far too woolly for someone as clearheaded as Simpson, and he immediately threw himself into denouncing the pseudo-science. The argument lasted some years, coming to an end when Simpson published in 1853 "Homeopathy, its tenets and tendencies", a scathing attack which sent the doctrine into disrepute, whence it is only now beginning to stir.

The originator of homeopathy, Samuel Hahnemann spent most of his life in Leipzig. His principle was that "like cures like". As Belladonna caused symptoms resembling scarlet fever, it was to be used to cure scarlet fever. Similar reasoning used cinchona for ague, and ipecacuanha for asthma. A rule of the system was that only one remedy was to be used at a time, and a second dose not to be given until the first had ceased to act. Also the dose was to be so small that it would only act on the disease, Hahnemann arguing that the smaller the dose, the greater its potency. He diluted and rediluted a solution of the drug again and again, stating that disease produced an abnormal sensitiveness. Even the smell of the drug was enough at times, provided the correct remedy had been chosen.

Naturally the new idea was strongly opposed by the apothecaries, who had grown rich on the once fashionable habit of prescribing bigger and better doses of more and more drugs, a practice said to have caused more deaths than the French Revolution and Napoleonic Wars put together.

Robert Christison describes homeopathy as "drops of nothingness, powder of nonentity and extractum nihile". Simpson's published pamphlet contained an extraordinary amount of information and its impact was immediate. One critical comment came from Ireland. "I cannot conceive any person not labouring under monomania who can read it without being convinced, but its size will be with many an excuse for not reading it all all! Is it worth trying to reason fools out of their folly?"

The most reputable doctors agreed that the technique was a system of "professional swindling". Professor Syme, who was said to treat all medicines with disdain and perhaps even all physicians, moved that anyone admitting to be a homeopathist should be disqualified by the Medical Chirurgical Society of Edinburgh. Simpson seconded the motion, and in a convincing speech to the Society urged the use of common sense.

Meanwhile, Simpson wrote a prodigious number of letters. His correspondence during the early 1840s is full of casual references that suddenly flared up into major rows, and his accounts include bills to John Robertson, his solicitor, for assessing libellous remarks.

D

Mr Robertson advised Simpson not to pursue yet another argument with Syme. The quarrel came to a head when both men met outside a patient's door, each having been called in by the family doctor, Dr Beilby who was at this time President of the College of Physicians. Syme took exception to Simpson's presence, accusing him of meddling in fields beyond midwifery, while Simpson retaliated by naming Syme as the writer of slanderous letters concerning his behaviour, which had recently been printed in a medical journal. The two men shouted at each other, oblivious of the flapping ears of the patient and retinue of subsidiary medical attendants; finally both stormed off.

Provided Simpson had the last word, which he usually did, he seemed prepared to forget the issue, but his antagonists were often too deeply hurt to do the same. To Simpson, a current argument was one of many, and, having underlined his point, he would switch his attention to something else. He was surprised that his colleagues did not do the same.

James Miller, an Edinburgh surgeon, was a good friend of Simpson. In 1842 the surgical chair became vacant and Miller applied for the post. Simpson vigorously supported him, until he discovered that Syme was also canvassing for Miller. Hastily, Simpson changed his allegiance to the opposing candidate, Lizers, raking up an unfortunate case in which a patient of Miller had died after an operation as an explanation for his sudden lack of confidence.

After the chair had been awarded to Miller, Simpson considered the matter closed and was most put out when his overtures of friendship were turned down. "A little cool reflection could convince even Simpson that I was hardly to be blamed," wrote Miller ruefully. "I could forgive and would forget, but self respect will not permit me to, and I must decline the extraordinary offer of renewed intimacy he makes, now that the canvass is over."

On reading the vast residue of correspondence, Simpson leaves the impression that his rows and feuds were good-natured, without malice, and that the acrimony is something of a façade. There is no account of him ever losing his temper, and it is not too much of a contrast for instance, to find that he can also write the most tender letters, such as this to his father-in-law, about his little daughter.

23rd December 1841

My dear Mr. Grindlay,

We are all well and hearty here and Maggie has just been before tea laughing and skirling at a great rate. She tries to walk by a hold, and appears to think herself mighty clever when she manages a few steps. I have been very busy in practice for several weeks past and often wish the day were 30 hours long in order to get all done that ought to be done. Yesterday I had the honour of waiting on several 'Hon' ladies, on three daughters of the Lord President, on Lady Dundas and in the evening on Lady Anstruther who had a nice little lively daughter after an hour or two only of real suffering.

I am using 2 horses—one for the day and the other for evening work.

Maggie often chuckles over her apple pie book and seems to admire most the part of "G—gobbled it".

Your affectionate son,
J. Y. Simpson.

Simpson's name was now well known among the Scottish members of the House of Lords, and this obviously helped to bring him such patients as Princess Marie of Baden, wife of the Duke of Hamilton. In fact, Simpson was by now one of the best known obstetricians in the country, and, like his collagues, in Europe, had become increasingly interested in operative gynaecology on the mother, as well as the delivery of the baby.

Women were beginning to demand and expect attention at other times than only during labour, and Simpson was the first doctor in Britain to offer them practical treatment and hope for a cure. As the procedures were new, instruments were lacking or inadequate, but Simpson was never stopped for lack of a tool. Medical historians give him the credit for the invention of the uterine sound, which is to this day used unaltered, and this great invention actually came about by accident. He was using an ordinary straight metal bougie one day, but dropped it on the floor. He stood on it, by mistake, which bent one end, and "Hey Presto, the uterine sound". He immediately realised that the instrument was now much more useful and used it for some time before publishing a description of it in the

Edinburgh Monthly Journal of Medical Science in June 1843. He never claimed it was original, for Hippocrates and Soranus had mentioned a similar instrument, but he was the first to use the sound "diagnostically for parts usually considered beyond the reach of examination".

Source of light was a major difficulty to medical practice in the 1840s, and operations were often postponed because "it was a cloudy day". Simpson liked to see what he was doing, and was still not satisfied with his access to the seat of gynaecological troubles, the uterus, or womb. His sound could tell much about the structure of the interior of the uterus, but he now turned his attention to exposing it so that it could actually be seen by opening it up in a manner similar to the natural process that takes place during labour. He announced success in a paper to the Medical Chirurgical Society in 1844, and described his technique to the audience. "For several years past I have been constantly employing this means of dilation of the uretic cavity for a variety of purposes and indications." His method was to insert a conical shaped sponge which had been steeped in gum arabic and compressed around a wire and held together by whip-cord. When moist, the sponge would expand, which it did when in position, so opening up the mouth of the uterus. It stayed in place by the spirally grooved surface resulting from the whip-cord. A series of tents, of increasing size, could be used, until adequate dilation was achieved. A well-made tent took twenty to thirty hours to expand fully a reflection on the length of time a Victorian doctor was prepared to spend on his patient and an explanation of why this method has been superseded!

In Burns's *Textbook of Midwifery*, the most enlightened handbook of the period, blood letting, purgation and opiates were the standard remedies to obstetrical problems and lubrication with lard a ready answer to the tedious labour. No wonder Simpson's waiting room was rather crowded with women desperate to consult someone whom they had heard was prepared to try something else. Maternal death rate at this time was 10 in 1,000. Often some quick manipulation would have saved mother or child, but the surgeon's hand was stayed by the reluctance of inflicting more agonies on the woman who, as it was, could hardly bear the pain. Obstetricians in Europe and the New World knew now that it was possible to open the abdomen and operate on various organs, and papers were being constantly read on increasingly adventurous advances on the patients' organs which would denfiitely cure their problems. But most surgeons hesitated to try out such barbarous cruelty on the wide awake woman at their mercy. Now, however, education was beginning to make the Victorian woman more aware of herself and not so ready to accept a bottle of medicine and a leech from a benevolent physician. Women of the middle and upper classes travelled about the Continent freely during the 1840s, and gossiped in their drawing rooms of many enlightened things, including obstetrics. Simpson's name crept up often and with devotion. As is apparent by reading their diaries numerous women realised that here was a man prepared to treat them as individuals with particular problems. Here were the first stirrings of the Womens' Liberation Movement and Simpson was championing their cause.

Simpson crystallises his own opinion and explains his attitude to the practice of Medicine at this time in an address that he was delighted to give to the newly qualified medical students in 1842. The medical faculty professors took it in turns to deliver the graduation address, in which they were expected to inspire the students with advice and words of wisdom on this last occasion that they were under the thumb of the University. When the rota came round to Simpson for the first time, he treated the event with great seriousness and devoted much time to his speech, in which he set down his own principles and ambitions. As was his habit, he then hastily printed it as a leaflet, which he circulated far and wide, thus making full use of the time spent on writing the miniature thesis.

In the address, he first warns the newly qualified doctors that they know nothing. "This day is the beginning of your professional studies, not the end." He points out that the professors have given them a foundation, but it is up to the men themselves to build the superstructure of their life by their own efforts.

The only way to professional distinction is by extending one's knowledge, and exploiting it to the full. The more one knows, considered Simpson, the greater is one's enthusiasm for the subject. Interest in a patient's disease must be greater than interest in his money, and then the rewards will be far greater than any cash value of a full wallet.

"In struggling towards fame and fortune, place from the first all hopes for advancement in your medical ability alone." Simpson warns them to have no illusions that patronage or wide social circles will increase their private practice. This will only lose time, and, what is worse, habits of indolence and indulgences will be substituted for habits of study and exertion. No one will entrust his life to another just because he is their friend, for "to have professional confidence in you, he must respect you as a doctor". Social success in the drawing room calls for quite different qualities than those longed for and valued in the sick room. Only a medical reputation will bring you patients. "The public will not employ you for your advantage and your interests, but for their advantage and their interests alone." There is no one so selfish as a sick man.

Simpson continues: "Every man has control of forming his own habits, so choose carefully, and teach yourself to save time. There are always minutes here and there that can be added together; never lull your mind into listless idleness. The busiest people are the ones who can always find time for something else. Keep your eye on your clock. Punctuality is the secret for getting things done. Have a duty for every time and you will have time for every duty."

Frittering away time is bad enough, emphasised Simpson, but, more important "never fritter away your thoughts". A good physician must be able to fix his mind at will and concentrate on the subject at hand to the exclusion of everything else. The difference between a genius and the rest, he contended is his ability to force himself to think. Isaac Newton claimed that any mental superiority that he had was purely due to this habit of mental application. Nothing comes to one easily, the rewards of life come only in proportion to effort spent. Go out and make opportunities, they never come to one sitting at home. Aim for the highest mountain, and strain every nerve to reach the top. We won't all get there, but we will do better than we otherwise would, and don't go under with difficulties; be stimulated by them instead. There is no such thing as luckless fate, it's just another word for apathy and mismanagement.

Passionate desire can perform impossibilities. Few obstacles stand up to a determined effort, and, as the horizon melts before the polar traveller, if one strives on, long enough, some path will always open up among the hills.

"Your aim is to alleviate human suffering, and gladden as well as prolong the course of human life. In this country, this light of benevolence will make you happy, but if you start working with a cold-hearted view to money, your life will be as dark and miserable as that low and grovelling lust that dictates it."

Simpson's final advice is for the young physician to "obey the rules. Stick to the ethics and etiquette observed by medical men. And, if it is possible, don't enter into arguments or throw out cantankerous remarks! Remember," he emphasised at the closing of the address, "Your future career is a matter of your own choice, not chance."

At present Simpson's own life was somewhat darkened with money troubles. Having lent all his new savings to a friend, he found himself badly in need of some ready cash. As he explained in a letter to Sandy asking for yet another loan,

Dr Hamilton's daughters last week sold the Lying-in-Hospital with all its furniture, beds, teacups, etc. I had to put £30 of furniture myself, which I was obliged to buy back on Thursday last from Mr Brown, the purchaser, with all the other things to put into a new hospital. The hospital is necessary for the class. We are ordered to flit tomorrow and have not yet got a house. I expect to get the use of the Fever hospital for a few weeks to put our poor patients in. Dr Hamilton would blush to see what his family have done. I must exert myself for some months to come to get a new hospital set a-going.

He was house-hunting on his own behalf just now too. Another child had arrived, and Simpson wrote to Mr Grindlay to invite him to the christening.

The little fellow thrives like a mushroom. Maggie has a go cart today and seems perfectly amazed at her own performances in walking in it. I wish very much to come down for other reasons. I have been looking at the outside of several houses for flitting farther West where my business is lying more and more. There are several in Charlotte Square and Queen Street and we would have a ramble through them all if you would only come down.

He urged Mr Grindlay to take the boat from Liverpool to the Clyde, then to use the new Glasgow Railway, which cut down the journey between the two cities to nearly one hour.

At this point in his life Simpson was full of enthusiasm and his letters to the family and friends overflow with exuberance and a boyish pride in his aristocratic patients. He bought a claret curricle and changed to two younger, friskier ponies which clattered over the cobbles between the Old and New Towns, swinging into the University Quadrangle, scattering the groups of students, and charging down the Mound in a flourish of colour and noise.

Then tragedy struck.

My dear Janet,

My own dear Maggie was taken from me this morning between 9 and 10 o'clock. She was attacked with measles 2 days ago and was subsequently seized with a very bad form of sore throat, which after several days struggle at last became worse on Friday morning and proved too strong and fierce for her little emaciated body. It was ultimately so heart rending to witness her terrible anxiety and restlessness that her demise was almost a relief to all of us. She asked for "a drink of water" for her little parched and burning throat a very short time before she died but then for hours before was unable to swallow it.

My dear Jessie has behaved herself well under the stunning blow and is better than I could have hoped for. Though dreadfully broken down she is submitting to our affliction with great fortitude.

My dear Maggie's life has been a short one and these first hours of grief look almost like a dream—but a dream I hope will leave behind it fond, fond fond recollections of her.

Breaking the news to his mother-in-law, Simpson writes:

Maggie is now stretched out in a white bed in the parlour.

Her eyes are quite open and she looks beautiful but still as if suffering. As we look at her it seems almost strange and unexplicable that she does not yet still breathe and move.

My own dear Jessie has behaved herself under this sad and stunning trial with the greatest propriety and fortitude but her mind is one which I fear will suffer longer and more deeply than many others. . . .

I have written a long long note absurdly so—but oh I hope you will excuse it under the circumstances for now that our dear Maggie has left us it is a source of pleasure of an indescribable kind to be allowed to talk of her even on paper.

The Simpson family had no burial site in Edinburgh, but James could now afford a family plot. He bought a stretch of green turf in Warriston Cemetery at Inverleith, on the northern side of the town. It is a peaceful place. The dark skyline of the Old Town "lands" and its spires, and the long rectangular shapes of the New, can be seen stark against a backdrop of the blurred folds of Arthur's Seat with the etched profile of the Salisbury Crags, and the gentle bulk of the Pentland Hills beyond; to the right is the Castle high on its rock, and visible most of the way to Bathgate.

Maggie's death left a deep scar. Years afterwards, a mention of her name led Simpson to describe her smile and winning ways. He was never quite so exuberant again. But life went on, and in February 1845 Simpson wrote to Mr Grindlay:

I purchased a house this morning in Queen Street. It lies between Castle Street and Frederick Street, has a fine public garden before it and a small one with stable and coach house behind. It has four more rooms for beds than our present one—and is a storey higher. It is not fashionably done up, but looks a good comfortable place. I only heard of it 48 hours ago—I had no intention of moving this year. The price is £2,150. The fee duty is about £5 yearly. It is probably the most central part of the town—and so far favourable. Nor is the price of property likely to decrease there. In fact it is rising higher and higher in Edinburgh. The dining room flat contains two back rooms and there are two drawing rooms and a bedroom in the second flat; four bedrooms in the third (one of them very large and an excellent nursery). The money is to be paid at Whit Sunday. I will have no difficulty in getting my own house let.

We are all well. Excuse haste and believe me, my dear Sir,
Your very affectionate son,
J. Y. Simpson."

Jessie Simpson begins to retreat into the background of her husband's life with their removal to Queen Street. She wrote to her mother soon after Maggie's death "I miss her all day, everywhere". Jessie was a complacent, resigned soul, and it is difficult to bring her into focus. She obviously had much to put up with, and perhaps her passivity was a good thing. One effervescent character in the family was quite enough.

Jessie had little attention from her husband at this time, for he was very busy amassing statistics for a paper on the frequency of death in hospital after an amputation, as compared with the greater chance of survival if the operation was carried out at home. This branching into the surgical field was a tactless gesture as far as his relationship with his old enemy Syme was concerned and threw them once more at each other's throats.

The fact was that two in three patients died after amputation of the thigh in Edinburgh Royal Infirmary, and Simpson had felt since students days that this proportion was too high. The paper that he published at this time did not offer a solution, but the question of hospital infection in general, and puerperal fever in particular was turning over in his mind, resulting in his great thesis on hospitalisation which appeared twenty years later.

In spite of his advice to the graduates never to cultivate patients, or mix social life with work, Simpson greatly enjoyed his sallies into aristocratic circles, as his letters reveal.

I was at Hamilton Palace last week seeing the Marchioness of Douglas. I have half promised to go to London to her in March. She pressed me to stay and have the honour of dining with the Duke of Cambridge. I preferred having the honour of *refusing* as Forbes Angus was waiting for me. . . .

In November I expect to bring into the World heirs to three Earldoms. Of course I calculate on the three youngsters being all boys. I all but agreed to make a visit to Lord and Lady Douglas at Brodick Castle and *try* to shoot grouse.

There is a quality among the Scots that makes them acceptable in a much higher stratum of society than that in which they were born. A Scot's tongue is an asset. Education is the criterion, not money or birth. Sir Walter Scott said, "There is a certain intuitive knowledge of the world to which most well educated Scotsmen are easily trained that prevents them from being much daunted by this species of elevation."

Simpson did go to London, and, as he pointed out himself, in rather different circumstances from his first visit to the capital ten years previously. News in the streets of London of Lady Blantyre's impending baby included a printed life of her Scottish obstetrician.

Simpson wrote to his sister-in-law.

Stafford House, London.

My dear Isabel,

As I have just risen from dinner I am not disposed just now for study, I will (provided you will allow me) scribble you a page—

I arrived here on Friday, and as I think, just in time, they were all very kind to me on my arrival, and my rooms look into St James' Park—with one of the prettiest views in London—Stafford House is situated between St James' and Buckingham Palace—thence in a most royal vicinity. The House itself is most magnificent—particularly the entrance Hall. The Hall is the whole height of the house—of enormous breadth as well as height, has a hanging stair on its sides of 20 more feet in width—its walls are from top to bottom solid and variagated marble broken with enormous pillars—and immense mirrors multiplying the effect of the whole. The stair and landings are covered—every inch of them—with red cloth and the balustrades and roof are deeply inlaid with gold. The whole looks a fairy scene—couches and chairs are thrown around the hall—stairs and landings—and the family seem sometimes to dine and drink tea in this part of the house. Lord Blantyre took me today through the drawing room and

picture galleries. The walls and roofs are ebony and gold—
and look magnificent. The family are all good, loveable plain
folks. We all dine all the hour of *two* (how unfashionable). Tea
at five or six—supper when you please—Today our dinner
party consisted of the Duke, Marquis of Stafford, Marquis
of Lorne, Lord Blantyre, Lady Lorne, Lady Constance
Gower, and Lord Lorne seems to me the *greatest* aristocrat of
the whole—but apparently is very sharp and clever. I did not
like him yesterday but I sat next to him today at dinner and
he talked and smoothed down wonderfully. Mr. Rasleigh the
M.P. for Cornwall, was on his other side. His wife went down
to Edinburgh two weeks ago to be under my care. Lady
Lorne is a very sweet, unaffected girl—and so is my patient.
The Duchess is sick and I had to prescribe for her today. She
seems very gentle and quite a domestic woman—her figure is
magnificent. The Duke is, in appearance, very like Dr Muir
of Edinburgh—and the resemblance seemed both to strike
and amuse Lord Lorne when I mentioned it at dinner today
—They all eat as fast as Americans. Our Dinner Table is a
round one filled with fruit in the centre and a few dishes
around the sides. All meats are brought from the side table.
The plates of silver—the potatoe dishes large plain Scotch
wooden "Cogues"—Our wines, port, sherry and claret—

I have been very happy since I came—1st because I have
plenty of time to give to my own beloved books and papers—
2nd because I am beginning to feel rested—and 3 because the
family are so kind as to put me quite at my ease.

My advent to London this time is certainly a very different
one from what it was 10 years ago. Yesterday I took a stroll
out and bought the enclosed life of me—published on the
day of my arrival. Is that ominous? I have been mightily
diverted by it and laughed till I was sore at the account of our
courtship. What will Jessie say?

Yours affectionately,
J.Y.S.

His new clientele, and visits to English Castles and Scottish
Keeps, must have had an effect on the drawing room in the
homely house in Queen Street. Simpson's eagle eye noticed
everything, and he relished a new experience. "I think now

artificial flowers very ungenteel," he wrote home after a visit to another titled patient.

> The ladies here wear nothing but real flowers in their hair—Rowans and haws are often worn beaded into crowns or chaplets. Heather is also a favourite. On Thursday Lady Lorne came down with a most beautiful chaplet tying round and keeping down her braided hair. It was a long bunch of bramble leaves and half ripe bramble berries—actually true brambles.
>
> I really feel quite at home among them—though the only untitled personage at the table.

Simpson's feet however, were kept firmly on the ground by his work at the Lying-in-Hospital, and by his friends. Dr Sharpey now a professor in the University College Hospital wrote from London that he must remember to acknowledge letters from General Practitioners and Christison sent a note round acidly reminding him to keep appointments. Another friend wrote,

> I must point out to you the reports which are everywhere current of your inattention to patients who place themselves under your care. That you neglect one set for the sake of another, that you break appointments, keep patients in their beds waiting for you day after day, that letters remain unanswered and that patients are often left in ignorance whether they are to alter, continue or give up the remedies you have prescribed.
>
> Now, excuse me for stating the absolute necessity for some change to be made.

Perhaps the patients would not have minded had they known what was filling Simpson's mind in 1847, and taking up his time well into the night.

CHAPTER VII

Ether

January 19th, 1847.

MY DEAR SANDY,

I believe you will be glad to hear that I am to be appointed one of her Majesty's Physicians in Scotland. . . . Flattery from the Queen is perhaps not common flattery, but I am far less interested in it than in having delivered a woman this week without any pain while inhaling sulphuric ether. I can think of naught else.

This successful use of ether was immediately submitted in a paper to the *Monthly Journal of Medical Science*. Simpson began the manuscript, with the following

Not poppy nor mandragora
Nor all the drowsy syrups of the world.
Shall ever medicine thee to such sweet sleep.

From earliest times attempts had been made to relieve pain by drugs. An Arab sheik introduced Indian hemp, which induced rapturous excitement and intoxication, bud did nothing to deaden the excruciating agony of the surgeon's knife. The Egyptians used opium as well as Indian hemp, and the Greeks and Romans the wine of mandragora and opium weed laced with alcohol. The Greeks also compressed the carotid artery in the neck, and had traced the practice to the Assyrians who made their young lads unconscious in this way before performing circumcision. St Mark says Christ was offered wine mingled with with myrrh before being nailed to the cross, and Helen gave Ulysses the same sort of drink which "wrapped the soul in night" in preparation for death. Soldiers of the Orient threw myrrh and wine on to hot stones and inhaled the fumes to quell the pain from their battle wounds.

Mandragora, the mandrake plant, had been used since time immemorial as a love potent, aprhodisiac and hypnotic. Salen of Greece used it to deaden pain, and Apelius claimed that half an ounce of mandragora taken with wine would induce such a deep sleep that a limb could be sawn off or burnt without causing any pain. The mediaeval doctors travelling with the Crusading armies used a "sleeping sponge" that was soaked with the juice of the Morel fungus, hemlock, lettuce, mulberry, poppy and mandrake, and was held to the nostrils of the wounded to deaden the pain of amputation. Warriors, gladiators and soldiers had been taken care of since early days; no one had thought of women. Letting blood to the point of fainting appeared to be the only remedy for relieving their pain. In 1805 a thesis appeared in America entitled "The means of moderating or relieving pain during parturition" which suggested that pain in childbirth must be regarded as a disease, having its origin in the changes produced by civilisation and refinement. Doctors had made no attempt to alleviate the agonies of childbirth because of the prevailing sentiment that pain in labour was inevitable and necessary. The only thing to do, the writer advised, was to let more blood.

From the dawn of history till the early nineteenth century pain was part of the experience of every pregnant woman and to a certain extent every man. The soporific sponges were not much good when it came to having one's leg sawn through. It was still a brutal age, when public executions were regarded as a form of entertainment, and the British Army branded its deserters with the letter D and flogged its troops. Boys of 6 were toiling in the coal pits and girls and young women working at the power looms from 6 in the morning to 7 at night, with a quarter of an hour off for breakfast and three quarters for lunch. A child of 8 would have no more time to play than would an adult and would be just as likely to have his limbs entangled in the whirling cogs of the new fangled machines. *The Lancet* reported as late as 1883 that a woman making trousers earned 1/– a day, for which she worked for 17 hours. The Americans were still buying and selling their slaves and the Boston Medical and Surgical Journal of 1845 records the case of a negress sold at full term pregnancy, who died of puerperal fever. Under the guarantee of soundness, it asks, ought the buyer or the seller be the loser?

In 1772 Sir Walter Scott's uncle, Daniel Rutherford, had discovered nitrogen gas, and in the same year Joseph Priestley came across nitrous oxide, "laughing gas". Humphry Davy followed up these investigations, but he was a chemist, not a doctor, and his experiments were purely for the laboratory. He inhaled the gas himself, and persuaded the poets Coleridge and Southey to do the same. He was well aware of the analgesic properties of the gas and suggested it could be used for surgical operations, but no doctor looked into the matter, and surgeons continued to operate on struggling patients held down by straps and strong men. Davy's most famous assistant, Michael Faraday, went farther and discovered sulphuric ether. In 1818 he wrote, "When the vapour of ether mixed with common air is inhaled it produces effects very similar to those occasioned by nitrous oxide. By the incautious breathing of ether vapour, a man was thrown into a lethargic condition which lasted for 30 hours."

A country doctor, Henry Hickman, was the first to realise that inhalation of a gas could enable him to operate on a patient who would feel no pain. He tried hard to bring his idea to public notice, printed papers, and even petitioned the King of France. The Royal Society was uninterested, and he died at thirty without recognition.

On breathing nitrous oxide, the patient is thrown into paroxysms resembling uncontrollable laughter. Long before it was used as an anaesthetic, the gas made its public appearance, on the music hall stage. In 1830 eighteen-year-old Samuel Colt was touring New England giving laughing gas exhibitions to raise money for the patenting of his revolver, which could produce more pain, through injury, than most earlier weapons put together.

Then in 1843 two young men arrived in Boston, U.S.A. to establish a practice in dentistry. One called Thomas Morton and the other Horace Wells. Boston was a prosperous city known to the Americans as the "Hub of the Universe". But success did not come as quickly as the partners felt it should. However, Morton was optimistic in the face of the empty dental chair. "You have to drive ahead in this age of steam," he is quoted as saying, "or you will be run over and no one will ever stop to pick you up." He realised that in order to draw in patients they needed a new and unique method of treatment to offer the public. The accepted method in Boston of preparing a mouth for false teeth was to knock off the crowns, leaving the roots, and over this hinge monstrosities made from hippopotamus tusks. Saliva soon changed these from bluish white to saffron yellow, with a black line around the margin of each tooth. Morton decided to do better than this, and set to work to find an alternative material to hippo tusk. He began to dabble in chemistry and found a substitute in felspar combined with metallic oxidies, which he enamelled by hand to look like teeth. At the same time he read a paper describing a new method of securing teeth in the mouth, called the "atmospheric suction principle". Morton's confidence soared, and he inserted a bold advertisement in the Boston Post on the front page, announcing his ability to make the "perfect set".

Wells, his partner was not so sure of success. In order to prepare the mouth for teeth that could be held in by atmospheric pressure they would have to extract the roots. No one did that in Boston. Wells was sure that the patient would refuse to endure the agony of this procedure. His courage collapsed and he withdrew from the partnership. The challenge was now Morton's and he set to work by himself. By February 1844, he was so successful that he had to add two assistants to his staff, and import 3,000 lbs of felspar in order to cope with the demand for his dazzling teeth.

Morton realised that there was only one thing that might undermine his secure and thriving world: the problem of pain. The screams from his patients as he wrenched with his dental forceps began to frighten him, and he stepped up his doses of whisky and laudanum. This helped very little and only made the ladies of Boston sick. Morton was suddenly very afraid that his success would be short lived and his dental practice a failure after all. He began to realise his ignorance. An answer to the problem of pain must lie in drugs, chemistry and medicine, and he was bitterly aware of his lack of knowledge in this wider field.

Morton resolved to become a doctor, and set to work to study

for the entrance qualificatins of the Medical School. He decided
to take some preliminary lessons in chemistry, and enrolled
himself as a student of a Dr Charles Jackson, who had already
helped him with a formula for soldering the felspar in the
making of his false teeth.

With Jackson, Morton discussed a distillation of chloric acid
and alcohol, known as chloric ether, which had been used for
some time as an inhalation for relieving asthma and other
breathing complaints. Accorging to Jackson, medical students
in Boston sometimes inhaled the fumes as a cheap way of
producing the effect of alcohol, and called these parties "ether
frolics". Jackson also told Morton that skin could be made
insensitive by sprinkling ether on the surface, and he gave
Morton some to try.

Morton now began his medical training. The leading surgeon in Boston was a Dr John Warren, whose influence went
much farther than the Massachusetts General Hospital, where
he worked. Morton received a letter from his old partner Wells,
who wrote to say that he had made a fantastic discovery: he
knew how to draw teeth without pain! He explained that he
had been very intrigued with a music hall demonstration of
nitrous oxide gas and had now learned how to make the gas
himself. He had used it on fifteen dental patients, not one of
whom had felt a twinge of pain. He wrote now to ask Morton to
arrange for a demonstration of the gas in Boston. Morton rushed
to Dr Warren, the leading surgeon, who agreed at once to
allow Wells to appear in front of his anatomy class. The evening
arrived, and Wells asked his patient to breath deeply from a
spigot attached to an india-rubber bag filled with nitrous
oxide gas. But the gas did not prove so reliable as Wells had
hoped. In a few seconds the patient appeared stupefied, and
trembling with excitement, Wells fixed his forceps on the tooth.
He started to pull—instanty the patient catapulted from his
chair, howling with pain. Pandemonium broke out in the lecture
theatre, as students began to hiss and stamp. Wells left Boston
next morning without seeing Morton again and turned his
attention to exhibiting birds and manufacturing showers.

A few weeks after this fiasco Morton, the medical student
watched Dr Warren amputate the leg of a man of 50. As Morton
looked on, he was appalled at the stark searing agony of the

man as he writhed and heaved on the table, strapped down and held by four hefty assistants, while the knife bit into his flesh. Morton wrote afterwards that it was at this moment, that he now realised his search and pre-occupation with pain killers had greater meaning than the saving of his dental practice.

During the summer of 1844, Moreton was faced with several dental patients who seemed particularly susceptible to pain. There was a Miss Parrot, whose tooth was so sensitive she could not bear Morton to touch it. As he waited for Miss Parrot to recover before he tried again, he considered the bottle of chloric ether which Jackson had given him a few months before. It crossed his mind that perhaps he could desensitise the tooth, as Jackson had suggested was possible on the skin. Morton poured some into the cavity of Miss Parrot's tooth, sealed it with wax, then waited one hour for effect. He then repeated the procedure twice.

His efforts were rewarded. "Doctor, I neither felt the instrument in the tooth, or your hand on my face, though I plainly see it in the mirror," Morton records Miss Parrot as saying.

Morton now turned all his attention to ether. He borrowed books from Jackson and picked the chemist's brain, all the while keeping the results of his experiments to himself. He inhaled ether combined with opium but the result was drowsiness and a headache. He then tried ether alone and breathed it from a handkerchief, which produced lassitude and numbness. He experimented with goldfish, birds and numerous insects, and discovered that he could control the ether easier if he combined it with "atmospheric air". Gradually he limited his experiments to himself and a large black spaniel, Nig.

Morton felt quite sure that he was moving in the right direction, He extended the time that he could put the dog to sleep, till, finally, it rebelled. Dodging Morton's hand one day, the dog's head hit the jar, knocking it over with a crash. Hastily Morton mopped up the escaping fluid with his handkerchief, and held it to his own nose. He continued breathing, the surroundings began to blur, and a deadening feeling came over him.

Boston, at that moment, was in an uproar. Congress declared war in Mexico and appropriated 10 million dollars to pay the initial cost. The New England states were up in arms in criticism. Boston was a stronghold of anti-slavery sentiment, and vehement speaches grew hotter and louder at the street corners, Quasi-religious temples and Revival Halls. Morton had another war on his hands too. His wife was expecting her second child and felt neglected. She wrote him tearful letters from her parent's house, threatening suicide. But Morton let nothing interrupt him now, and put all his concentration on making an apparatus for inhaling the ether and air.

As Morton worked out the final details of his experiment before actually trying it on his patients, he became increasingly cautious and secretive. He even bought his ether from various shops so that no questions would be asked as to the quantity that he was getting through. One difficulty though, kept cropping up. The quality of ether. Morton realised he needed advice. Reluctantly he turned again to the moody Dr Jackson, who at this time was involved in a legal battle as to who had invented guncotton. He insisted that he had, but he lost his case to an other.

Jackson was prepared to discuss the different preparations of ether on the market, and did not seem particularly concerned with what Morton intended to do with it.

By the evening of 30 September, Morton felt ready to try to anaesthetise a patient. He called his dental assistant over to their surgery and the two men were considering who to involve as a guinea pig, when the front door bell rang. On the doorstep was a large man, Eban Frost, clutching a swollen face. He said he was far too frightened and sore to have the tooth out, unless perhaps Dr Morton could mesmerise him. Morton said he could do better than that. He saturated a handkerchief in ether and held it over Frost's face. The patient greedily breathed in, and lost consciousness. Morton picked up his forceps and extracted the tooth. The patient neither moved nor woke up. The seconds lengthened. He still did not wake up. Morton threw water at him, shook him, and eventually dropped him. At that the patient gasped and opened his eyes. Morton pointed to the tooth on the floor. "No!" cried the man incredulously. "Glory Hallelujah!"

The next day the *Boston Daily Journal* carried the news and the dental practice was flooded with patients. Morton now wanted to go farther and administer his ether to one of Dr

Warren's patients in the Massachusetts General Hospital.

Dr Warren was sixty-eight. He was at the top of the surgical profession in America. His reputation was established. He was even known in European medical circles, and his papers were read in Britain and France.

Warren was susceptible to Morton's enthusiasm. He had always wished for a pain killing agent, and had permitted various demonstrations in the past, although all results had proved unsatisfactory and indefinite. He supposed he could allow one more demonstration. He said to Morton that when an opportunity came, he would allow him to bring his agent into the operating theatre of the Massachusetts General Hospital, and show what he could do.

Morton rushed off to prepare for the promised trial. He continued to etherise patient after patient in his dental surgery, perfecting his technique, and spent his evenings improving the inhaler. He drew sketches of one to be made in heavy glass, round in shape, the size of a man's head. Inside the mouthpiece were valves, or lips, which would open when the patient breathed in, close when he breathed out, thus retaining the ether in the globe. He took these drawings to an instrument maker in Boston, who promised to make an inhaler in a few days.

On 14 October Morton received a letter summoning him to the Massachusetts General Hospital on the following Friday 16th at 10 o'clock. He went into a frenzy of excitement, rushing to the instrument maker, altering the design of his inhaler, checking the purity of his ether, feeling that everything depended on the success of his performance at the hospital.

Eban Frost had agreed to go with Morton to the hospital, as living proof that the inhalation was harmless. Early on the Friday morning, the two men went to collect the instrument to find the maker with it still in pieces! Morton paced the floor in panic while it was reassembled, and rushed to the hospital ten minutes late.

The patient was a thin tubercular boy of twenty called Abbot; on the left side of his neck he had a large vascular tumour. Promptly at ten o'clock Dr Warren and a large retinue of Boston doctors approached the operating chair. Morton had not arrived. Dr Warren waited for five minutes, then solemnly raised his knife. At that instant a dishevelled Morton arrived, clutching his inhaler and jar of ether.

Restlessly everyone waited while Morton poured the ether into the inhaler, adding Eau de Mille Fleurs to cover the smell. He adjusted the mouthpiece, and put it between Abbot's lips. A high colour rose in the boy's pale cheeks. He seemed intoxicated. He mumbled and muttered and his limbs jerked convulsively.

Morton gave him more ether and he appeared to go to sleep. Dr Warren now went ahead. There was no cry of pain, no protest from Abbot as the knife cut into the growth on his neck. Warren calmly cut out the tumour and sewed up the wound. Slowly then, Abbot opened his eyes. "Have you felt pain?" demanded Warren. "I have experienced no pain," replied the boy, "Gentlemen," said Warren turning to the doctors and surgeons in the room "This is no humbug."

It was not until the later part of November that word of the properties of ether began to circulate outside Boston. The American medical journals were especially cautious with reference to new discoveries, and it took two months for the discovery to cross the Atlantic: in December 1846, however ether was administered in Paris and London.

Morton had won the world's battle with pain. His own personal battle had hardly begun.

Morton did not discover ether, others were working along the same lines, but he made ether anaesthesia known the world over and for that, merits all credit for the great achievement, and the honour should belong to him. As is inevitable in a scientific "discovery", many people were responsible for the eventual promotion of ether as an anaesthetic agent. Over 20 years previously Dr Hickman had proved that he could abolish surgical pain. Morton, however, had been prepared to go farther, and it was he who succeeded in making the world accept the discovery of anaesthesia, and bringing it out of the laboratory to every patient lying on the operating table, waiting the plunge of the surgeon's knife.

Morton was in America, where money and medicine go hand in hand. This was his downfall. He took out a patent on his "soporific agent", which he called "Letheon". Doctors were to pay him a fee before they could use it. Dr Jackson appeared on the scene again and claimed that the idea had been his and that he was therefore entitled to any money and credit for the great discovery. This was not the first time that Jackson had staked a thin claim: apart from the guncotton, he once said that it was he and not Mr Morse who had invented the telegraph! Wells reappeared too, and insisted that he was the true discoverer, not anyone else at all. Dr Jackson eventually went mad, Wells committed suicide and Morton died embittered and impoverished in 1868. But as Oliver Wendell Holmes said in America at the time "By this priceless gift to humanity, the fierce extremity of suffering has been steeped in the waters of forgetfulness and the deepest furrow in the knotted brow of agony has been smoothed for ever."

Morton's champions, Dr Warren and Dr Biglelow, saw to it that copies of the *Boston Journal* of 18 November were shipped to Europe. The news was also in letters on the Cunarder's wooden paddle steamer, *Acadia*, that arrived in Liverpool on 16 December.

The doctor on the *Acadia* was a Dr Fraser and when the ship berthed in Liverpool, he immediately set off home for Dumfries. There he saw his friend Dr Scott. He told him of the painless operations on sleeping patients in Boston, and 2 days later, 19 December, Dr Scott tried the idea out himself in the Dumfries and Galloway Infirmary. On the very same day, a Dr Boott anaesthetised a girl while a tooth was extracted in London by the same means and with the same successful results.

Dr Boott was actually born in Boston, although his mother was a Scot. He returned to graduate in Edinburgh, then practised in London, but made numerous voyages across the Atlantic and had many friends in America, and particularly Boston. That is why he received a letter from Dr Biglelow, written on 28 November with the account of the new process, all credit for which Biglelow gave to Morton. Dr Boott lived in Gower Street and with the help of a dentist neighbour they extracted a Miss Lonsdale's impacted molar tooth in Boott's study, his wife and daughters looking on in amazement.

On that same Saturday, Dr Boott delivered a note to London's leading surgeon, Robert Liston whom he had known from his Edinburgh days. Liston at once took action, and on the Monday tried it out for himself.

On 21 December 1846, at 2.25 on a wintery afternoon, Liston the son of the Ecclesmachan Manse, Linlithgow, announced to a full house of doctors and students that he was about to try a new invention that would render the patient insensitive to the knife that was to amputate his leg. Among the packed audience was a young man—Joseph Lister—as incredulous as the rest.

The patient was a butler, Frederick Churchill, and he was duly laid on the table, and quickly anaesthetised by Peter Squire. Twenty-eight seconds later the job was done. Churchill then started to struggle, protesting that he couldn't face the ordeal after all, and begged to be taken back to bed.

Liston turned to his audience, so excited that he stuttered, "This—this Yankie dodge, gentlemen, beats mesmerism hollow."

The lay press took little account of this historic happening, but the *Lancet* was enthusiastic. "That its discoverer should be an American is a high honour to our American brethren; next to the discovery of Franklin, it is the greatest contribution of the New World to Science."

While America squabbled about who, how and why ether had been discovered, Europe got on with using it. Dr Boott wrote to the Lancet saying that he had asked the Council's opinion, and that Morton's patent was invalid. No one on this side of the Atlantic seems to have given it another thought, and it was completely disregarded.

Simpson was always on to something new. Liston had written to Simpson's next door neighbour, James Miller, immediately after operating on the sleeping Churchill, and there is no doubt that Miller told Simpson the great news before reading this letter out to his surgical class on 23 December, only two days after the London occasion.

It was an enthusiastic letter announcing that "a new light had burst on Surgery, and a large boon conferred on mankind".

Simpson went to London himself at the tail end of the year. He wrote to Sandy that he had "breakfasted with the Secretary of War, dined with the Mistress of the Robes and had tea and an egg with the Premier. I went to see all the crack doctors at an evening discussion Society and found some of them busy speaking against my published opinions. I was driven to speak in self defence and set them right. I was a curious coincidence my popping in upon them at the time." Simpson also saw his old friend Liston and obviously got a first-hand account of the great event. He had always been a close student of the history of anaesthesia and knew all about the soporific sponge and artery compressions of the older days. He often remarked on their uselessness. He had nearly turned away from medicine when he had watched Liston crudely amputate the breast of a Highland woman many years before.

He was not the only one! Charles Darwin, while a student of Medicine at Edinburgh in 1828 relates how he "attended on two occasions the operating theatre and saw two bad operations, one on a child, but I rushed away before they were completed. Nor did I ever attend again for hardly any inducement could have been strong enough to make me do so. This being long before the blessed days of chloroform. The two cases fairly haunted me for many a long year."

Simpson at that time was quoted as saying "Can nothing be done to make operations less painful?" He had asked himself this question many times again. His contempories suppressed their feelings at their patient's agony. As Simpson said "the surgeon could bear the patient's pain no doubt somewhat easier than the patient". Speed was all they could offer the patient faced with an operation. America's leading obstetrician Charles Meigs declared that actually pain did a woman a lot of good. "Notwithstanding I have seen so many a woman in the throes of labour, I have always regarded a labour pain as a most desirable salutary and conservative manifestation of life force." He had no danger, of course, of experiencing this himself. Simpson was no ruthless surgeon; his soft hearted benevolence and kindliness has been mentioned time and again, and he had tried the various methods of relieving pain as they cropped up. He had turned his attention to mesmerism in 1837, when it was much in vogue, and had a lengthy correspondence with a Scottish doctor, James Esdaile, who seemed to have great success with the idea in Calcutta. He reported 261 painless operations. Indians perhaps were more receptive to the waving hands and suggestions of sleep, because in Europe the method was discredited and was treated as rather a joke by the practising surgeons whose patients still writhed under the knife.

Simpson found that he could influence a gullible patient to a surprising degree, and the polite New Town of Edinburgh was rife with alleged incidents of patients left in a trance while Simpson went out to the country. He tried his magic with toothache and sleeplessness, but could take it no farther than that.

But now, Christmas 1846, Simpson rushed back from London, fired with enthusiasm. It had been established that ether would induce anaesthesia for a surgical operation, which at this time lasted for a matter of moments; to put to sleep a woman in labour was another matter. The problems to be faced were quite different from those of the surgeon. Would the uterine contractions stop, thus simply postponing the mother's agonies? Would she develop the dreaded "convulsions of pregnancy"? What would happen to the baby?

As Simpson said at the time, "his mind was fully occupied with the thought", He wrote to Morton in Boston congratulating him on his great boon to mankind; and he received a letter giving accounts of the Dumfries operations. He does not appear, however, to have had any correspondence with the Professor of Obstetrics at Harvard. This American, Dr Walter Channing, was thinking along the same lines as Simpson, and which of the two professors first administered ether to the woman in labour is not known. Channing did not publish his account till 1848, but he states then that his experience "covered many years".

As far as Simpson and Europe was concerned, ether was first administered for the pain of labour when he gave it on 19 January 1847. He did not know what would happen. The woman had a contracted pelvis. Her first labour had been long and difficult and had lasted for four days. The child had eventually been drawn out in pieces, the operation taking more than an hour. She was the patient of a Mr Figg, who called Simpson to see her at 5.00 p.m., and again at 7.00. At 9.00 he decided to administer ether.

As she afterwards informed us, she almost immediately came under the anodyne influence of the ether, but in consequence of doubts upon this point its use was continued for nearly 20 minutes before I proceeded to turn the infant, as I had previously predetermined to do. A knee was easily seized and the child's extremities and trunk readily drawn down, but extreme exertion was required in order to extract the head. At length it passed the contracted brim. . . . The infant gasped several times but full respiration could not be established. On questioning the patient after the delivery she declared that she was quite unconscious of pain during the whole period, and her first recollection on waking was hearing but not feeling the head of the infant "jerk" from her. . . . She quickly regained full consciousness and talked with gratitude and wonderment of her delivery and her insensibility to the pains of it. Next day I found her very well in all respects. I looked in upon her on the 24th, the 5th day after delivery and was astonished to find her up and dressed and she informed me that on the previous day she had walked out of her room to visit her mother.

Simpson was delighted with this result and he started to use ether quite freely in his practice. France followed suit in a difficult forceps delivery on 30 January.

A patient's account of her experience gives a vivid picture of Simpson's state of mind at this time.

It was on a cold Sabbath night, in a villa near Blackford Hill, 28th February 1847, that he entered quickly, after midnight, to find that he was too late "I am so sorry" he whispered; "Why did not you send sooner? They said there was no haste. I told the man that I was to be out all night and that he must take me first to the Grassmarket, where a poor woman was lying very ill. When I could leave her and got to the foot of the stairs, the cab was gone, and I could only run out here. The man had thought I was to be all night with the poor woman." As he spoke he drew out of his pocket from under the folds of his winter coat a bottle of ether. ·'I'm so sorry, but you will never have to suffer such pain again. This would have put you to sleep and made it painless. I'll be out in the morning. Sleep now." His locks were pressed together with perspiration from his hard walk and his dark eyes kindled with regret and tenderness. . . . Long after he had disappeared the strange figure seemed still standing there, yet restless to go.

Simpson's attitude to the whole question of pain in child-birth is summed up in a paper published in March:

> Custom and prejudice and perhaps the idea of its inevitable necessity, make both the profession and our patients look upon the amount and intensity of pain encountered in common cases of natural labour as far less worthy of consideration than in reality it is. Viewed apart, and in an isolated light, the degree of actual pain is as great if not greater than that attendant upon most surgical operations. . . . The question which I have been repeatedly asked is this—shall we ever be justified in using the vapour of ether to assuage the pains of natural labour? . . . I believe the question will require to be quite changed in character. . . . It will become necessary to determine whether on any grounds, moral, or medical, a professional man could deem himself justified in withholding it.

Little did Simpson realise with what intensity this question would be asked at a later date, and that it would be left to him alone to find an answer.

The March paper on ether was widely circulated and the Berlin Obstetrical Society made Simpson an honorary member on the strength of it.

CHAPTER VIII

Chloroform

As 1847 ADVANCED, Simpson used ether in all his cases at the Lying-in Hospital and in his practice, administering it for a few minutes to start with, then up to several hours; but he was not entirely satisfied. Ether needed a heavy large glass bottle which was a nuisance to carry up and down the tenement stairs in the Old Town, and it had an objectionable smell that hovered over the patient long after it had been used, and made the ladies of the New Town sick. It was inclined to irritate the eyes, and a great deal was needed when used in a prolonged case of difficult labour. It also tended to catch fire if it was held too near the naked gas light. Simpson devised a special inhaler for using it, trying to improve its application, and wrote around the country for other people's impressions and results.

One letter out of hundreds, was to a Dr Fleming in Secunderabad.

I have sent you a short paper on ether. All here use it in surgical operations, and no doubt in a few years, its employment will be general over the civilized world. . . . The great secret of its exhibition is giving a large full and rapid dose of it at once. With many other medical men, I have taken it myself to try its effects. It is the only way of judging it.

During the summer and autumn of 1847 the surgical world slowly took to the use of ether, but doubts about its safety were beginning to be voiced. A letter from London states, "People here and in Paris are getting frightened of it, as the arterial blood becomes black under its influence and a few deaths have occurred."

Simpson paid little attention to the rumours, but he felt sure that there must be other gases capable of producing the "suspended animation" of ether. He wanted something more stable, quicker to act, easier to handle, and, being a practical man, something more portable.

Simpson was no scientist. He had no laboratory of cages of experimental animals. His dogs were part of the family and slept on his bed. With characteristic energy he looked round for his answer, and used the rough and ready method of inhaling any new fumes himself. After the day's work, he would produce the samples and set about trying them out. Jessie records two occasions when she found him unconscious on the basement floor in Queen Street. Simpson's neighbour, Professor Miller, records that "these experiments were performed at late night or early morn, when the greater part of mankind were soundly anaesthetised in common sleep!" During the autumn, Miller would look in to No. 52 every morning to see if there had been any success. Obviously he was prepared to forget his old grudge against Simpson.

The Professor of Chemistry, Lord Playfair, referred to one of Simpson's experiments in his memoirs.

On one occasion he came into my laboratory to ask whether I had any new substance likely to produce anaesthesia. My assistant, Dr Guthrie, had just prepared a volatile liquid, bibromide of ethylene, which I thought worthy of experiment. Simpson who was brave to rashness in his experiments, wished to try it upon himself in my private room. This I absolutely refused to allow, and declined to give him any of the liquid unless he promised me first to try its effects on rabbits. Two were procured, and under the vapour quickly passed into anaesthesia, coming out of it in due course. Next day Simpson proposed to experiment upon himself and his assistant with this liquid, but the latter suggested that they should first see how the rabbits had fared. They were both found to be dead! This has always appeared to me to be an excellent argument for experiments on living animals. By the sacrifice of two rabbits the life of the greatest physician of his time had probably been spared.

Assisting Simpson in his practice at this time were Drs George Keith and J. Matthews Duncan. Duncan was twenty, from Aberdeen. He had been influenced by Simpson to concentrate on obstetrics when attending his classes, and he had just returned from working in Paris when he joined Simpson in 1847. George Keith was the son of a Kincardine Manse, and he had travelled extensively in the Near East before working with Simpson. His young brother John was an apprentice to the practice at this time—one of the last doctors in Scotland to receive a clinical training in this time-honoured way. Simpson seemed to attract men of ability and these three were ultimately to de outstandingly well in their profession.

It was impossible for the three assistants to be near Simpson and not become involved in the search for an alternative gas to ether. They all took part in the experiments, sniffing at saucers of acetone, nitric ether, benzine. chloride of hydro carbon, the vapour of iodoform and many others, most of which they obtained from the University laboratory of Dr Gregory, or from Robert Christison who was particularly interested in drugs, mostly poisonous!

A Liverpool chemist from Simpson's student days visited 52 Queen Street in October, and suggested that pure chloroform might be suitable for his purpose. He was David Waldie, from Linlithgow, who had known Simpson in their student days, Waldie graduating in 1831. His main interest lay in chemistry and in 1840 he gave up medicine to become chemist to the Liverpool Apothecaries Company. There is no evidence to show if Simpson maintained contact with Waldie during his numerous visits to the seaport to see his wife's relations.

Waldie had worked with chloroform for Dr Formby, a Liverpool physician who had used it since 1838 in a diluted form as a stimulant and also as a soothing antispasmodic. Waldie had dissolved it in a known quantity of spirit, and so produced chloric ether of uniform strength. He promised now to prepare some pure chloroform for Simpson as soon as he returned to Liverpool and would send it up for trial.

Chloroform was a "curious liquid", first described by two chemists independently in 1831 and 1832. Its chemical and physical composition was first accurately determined by a distinguished French scientist, Dumas, in 1835. In 1842 Dr Mortimer Glover, a young Edinburgh graduate, discovered that it was a powerful narcotic posion to animals and that one of its effects was to produce insensibility. In early 1847 another

Frenchman, the physiologist Flourens, proved that inhaling it had the same effect as that of ether. Simpson had known since 1845 of Formby's use of the drug, but he said later that he did not know of Flourens' work. Because of Glover's research he had thought the drug sounded too dangerous and had up till now dismissed it.

Matthews Duncan mentioned chloroform again to Simpson in November and, as the promised sample had not arrived from Waldie in Liverpool because his laboratory had gone up in smoke, Simpson asked the local chemist, Duncan and Flockhart, to make him some. This arrived at 52 Queen Street, but it did not look very hopeful and the bottle was put aside.

Matthews Duncan had meanwhile been carrying out some research of his own. He had visited Dr Gregory's laboratory at the University and had carried off haphazardly a sample of every liquid in the laboratory that he imagined "would breathe". Chloroform was one of these. He knew nothing of Waldie's conversation with Simpson over this drug, and he told Robert Christison later, that one forenoon he tried out his collection with no results till he came to the chloroform. After ohe tentative sniff, he felt that here was something hopeful.

That very evening the three doctors gave the drug a thorough testing. Professor Miller was one of the first to hear of what happened, and he wrote his account soon after.

On returning home after a weary day's labour, Dr Simpson, with his two friends and assistants, Drs Keith and J. Matthews Duncan, sat down to their somewhat hazardous work in Dr Simpson's dining room. Having inhaled several substances, but without much effect, it occurred to Dr Simpson to try a ponderous material, which he had formerly set aside on a lumber-table, and which, on account of its great weight, he had hitherto regarded as of no likelihood whatever. That happened to be a small bottle of chloroform. It was searched for, and recovered from beneath a heap of waste-paper. And, with each tumbler newly charged, the inhalers resumed their vocation. Immediately an unwonted hilarity seized the party; they becmae bright eyed, very happy, and very loquacious, expatiating on the delicious

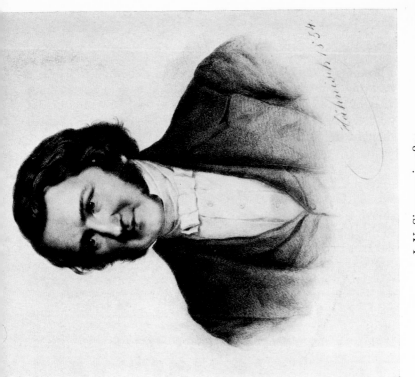

J. Y. Simpson in 1854

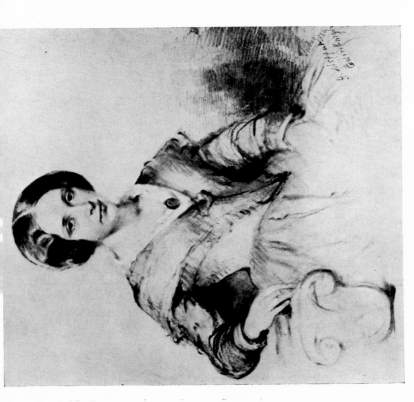

Jessie Grindley, 1846

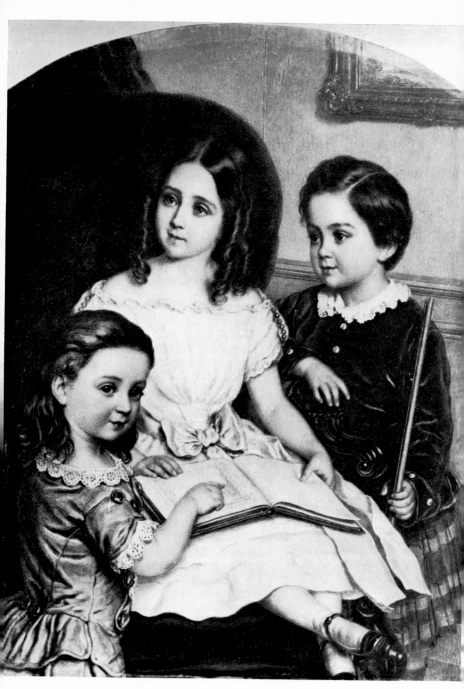

Three of the Simpson children
Magnus, Jessie and Wattie

aroma of the new fluid. The conversation was of unusual intelligence, and quite charmed the listeners—some ladies of the family and a naval officer, brother in law of Dr Simpson. But suddenly there was a talk of sounds being heard like those of a cotton mill, louder and louder; a moment more, then all was quiet, and then—a crash. On awakening, Dr Simpson's first perception was mental: "This is far stronger and better than ether," said he to himself. His second was, to note that he was prostrate to the floor, and that among the friends about him there was both confusion and alarm. Hearing a noise, he turned round and saw Dr Duncan beneath a chair, his jaw dropped, his eyes staring, his head bent half under him, quite unconscious, and snoring in a most determined and alarming manner. More noise still, and much motion. And then his eyes overtook Dr Keith's feet and legs, making valorous efforts of overturn the supper table, or more probably, to annihilate everything that was on it—I say, more probably, for frequent repetitions of inhalation have confirmed, in the case of my esteemed friend, a character of maniacal and unrestrainable destructiveness, always under chloroform, in the transition stage. By and by, Dr Simpson having regained his seat, Dr Duncan having finished his uncomfortable and unrefreshing slumber, and Dr Keith having come to an arrangement with the table and its contents, the *sederunt* was resumed. Each expressed himself delighted and with this new agent, and its inhalation was repeated many times that night—one of the ladies gallantly taking her place and turn at the table—until the supply of chloroform was fairly exhausted.

By this time it was 3.00 a.m. Simpson's guests were even more impressed than the three medical men. It took a lot to impress Simpson's brother-in-law, Captain Petrie, who was there watching with Jessie's sister and niece. The adventurous Petrie had been born in Fife in 1789, and Simpson and he had married sisters, the Grindlay girls of Liverpool. Simpson enjoyed the company of Captain Petrie, whom he had nearly served under, as ship's surgeon on the *Betsy*. Petrie had seen much action against the French in early years of the century, and was involved in the capture of Martinique and Guadeloupe, sailing

E

out from St Lucia, with 52 ships of the line, across the sparkling Carribean. He also served thoroughout the campaign against America after President Madison declared war with Great Britain in 1812. As a junior officer he led a detachment of his men to assist in the burning of the Capitol in Washington, in 1814. He grabbed a leather bound book of poetry from the library shelves before the flames took over, then sat down and finished President Madison's meal that he had abandoned to make his escape. The building had to be repainted after this, to cover the scars of the fire, following which it was always referred to as the "White House". Captain Petrie, Simpson's brother-in-law, insisted on taking away with him a bottle of the magic drug, so that he could invite guests to his home to have a sniff. His party was said to have been a great success, and the after effects not nearly as bad as rum!

The "gallant lady" referred to by Professor Miller was the family niece, Agnes Petrie. She had gone to bed on that important evening, after an early tea, but, hearing the extra-ordinary sounds from the dining room, had come down to investigate. She persuaded her uncle Simpson to let her join in, and he duly poured some of the drug into a saucer for her. She was somewhat large and fat, but the chloroform apparently had the marvellous effect of letting her slip out of her big body, and with an ethereal look on her podgy face she folded her hands on her chest and slid to the floor, crying out in extasy, "I'm an angel, oh, an angel". Her aunt Wilhelmina Grindlay did not dare to make such an exhibition of herself, and to the end of her long life refused to inhale chloroform. She said she never forgot the ghastly expression on Dr Keith's face as he eventually stopped kicking the heavy table, raised himself to his knees, his head level with the mahogony top, and stared wildly, straight at her. Simpson later used to tease her, chasing her with a bottle till she hid in a cupboard. She always escaped, for, to use Simpson's daughter's words, "fits of laughter used to seize him and choke him off the pursuit".

Another niece of Simpson's, Janet, stayed much at 52 Queen Street about this time, before marrying the Reverend James Wells of Pollokshields, Glasgow. After the wedding he discovered that his new bride had acquired the habit of whiffing herself into insensibility with a little chloroform before she went to sleep, and the first task the minister had to perform as a husband was to cure her of this very pecular habit!

Simpson was now absolutely confident that he had the answer. Chloroform appeared to have all the virtues. His experiments had proved that it had a rapid, easy induction, it was powerful and pleasant, easy to give, convenient and cheap It was non-inflammable and so could be given in small pokey rooms, near the fire or spouting gas jet. Simpson launched it on the world at once.

On 8 November he first used it on an obstetrical case. The patient was a doctor's wife, Jane Carstairs. She had recently returned from India, to live in Fife, but as she was expecting a difficult delivery, she moved across the Forth to Edinburgh and was staying at 19 Albany Street until the baby was born.

Jane Carstairs' last child had been born dead after a terrible labour lasting three days that ended with the baby's head being broken up before it could be extracted. However, for this her second confinement she consulted Simpson. Three hours after her pains started, he gave her chloroform. As he states in his "Notice of a New Anaesthetic Agent",

By moistening, with $\frac{1}{2}$ a teaspoonful of the liquid a pocket handkerchief rolled up into a funnel shape. . . . In consequence of the evaporation of the liquid it was once more renewed in about 10 or 12 minutes. The child was born in about 25 minutes after the inhalation had begun. The mother subsequently remained longer, I think stuporose, than commonly happens after ether. The squalling of the child did not arouse her; and some minutes elapsed after the placenta was expelled, and after the child was removed by the nurse into another room, before the patient awoke. She then turned and observed to me that she had enjoyed a very comfortable sleep and indeed required it as she was so tired (in consequence of extreme anxiety at the unfortunate result of her previous confinement she had slept little or none for 1 or 2 nights preceding the commencement of her present accouchment) but would now be more able for the work before her. I evaded entering into conversation with her, believing as I do that the most complete possible quietude forms one of the principal secrets for the successful employment of ether or chloroform. In a little time she again remarked that she was afraid her "sleep had stopped the pains". Shortly afterwards when the baby was brought in by the nurse from the adjoining room it was a matter of no small difficulty to convince the mother that the labour was entirely over and that the child presented to her was really "her own living infant".

The child was a girl, and her birth registered in Fife, for 9 November. She was christened on Christmas Day, 1847. Wilhelmina. Simpson sentimentally kept in touch with this child, and was sent a photograph of her at seventeen taken by a friend, John Adamson, a pioneer in photography. Because of her pious expression, Simpson jokingly named the study "St Anaesthesia", and always kept it above his desk.

Simpson read this account to the Edinburgh Medico Surgical Society on 10 November and his first written pamphlet appeared on the 15th. There is a footnote in this pamphlet, in which Simpson thanks Mr Waldie for first mentoining chloroform among other drugs as worthy of a trial, and also thanks Dr Keith and Dr Duncan for "the great zeal with which they have constantly aided me in conducting the inquiry".

A footnote acknowledgement of Waldie's part in the chloroform experiment was omitted from the acoccunt reprinted in the current medical journals, and his relations, at a much later date, took exception to this. But Waldie was only one of a number of chemists that Simpson consulted, and he had not been to produce the drug as promised

Simpson sent Waldie a copy of his pamphlet on 14 November with this covering letter.

My dear Sir,

I send you the first of the enclosed papers which I have myself sent off. My wife sent two, yesterday, one I think to Dr Petrie. I am sure you will be delighted to see part of the good results of our hasty conversation. I think I will get hold yet of some greater thing in the same way.

I had the chloroform in the house for several days before trying it as, after seeing it such a heavy unvolatile like liquid, I despaired of it and went on dreaming about others.

The first night we took it, Dr Duncan, Dr Keith and I all tried it simultaneously and were all under the table in a minute or two.

I write in great haste, as I wish to scribble off several letters.

Yours truly,
J. Y. Simpson.

Waldie, of course, would be envious that he had not investigated chloroform himself, but there is no evidence that he conducted any experiments on his own before Simpson told him of his results. Waldie's first publication on the subject of pain and chloroform was published in the *Lancet* on 1 January 1848, and after that his interest in chloroform appears to have faded out for the next twenty-two years, during which time he was making a fortune in Calcutta. On Simpson's death, however, the subject cropped up again, and in 1913 a plaque was erected to Waldie in Linlithgow, his birthplace.

Any surviving association Jackson or Waldie have with the history of anaesthesia is surely due to their luck in association with Morton or Simpson. If Simpson made no more mention of Waldie, what credit did Waldie give to M. Flourens, whose report on the anaesthetic properties of chloroform was read to the French Association of Science on the previous 8 March! Simpson was a tremendous worker, and in a hurry. He was thinking not of himself or of Waldie, but of chloroform. Under the circumstances, Waldie was lucky in that even his name remains.

Simpson is said to have been the midwife of the anaesthetic scene; he now had the infant in his hands and it was up to him to see it grow.

Satisfied that chloroform was suitable for his midwifery practice, Simpson was anxious to try it out in Surgery and turned to his next door neighbour Professor James Miller for an opportunity, and Miller was as keen to give it a try.

As we have seen Miller and Simpson had had many ups and downs in their relationships. Miller was the son of an Angus Manse, handsome and sensitive and an eloquent speaker. He had been a pupil of Liston and had the same bold approach to his work, but was said to break out in a sweat before he operated, always concerned about the pain he was to inflict and was known by his students as "the surgeon who hated to operate". He had paid great attention to Simpson's search for something superior to ether, and was the first to know of the successful evening of 7 November. All previous arguments between the two men were forgotten in Miller's enthusiasm for Simpson's new drug.

A few days later, 9 November, a patient with a strangulated hernia was brought into the Royal Infirmary. Miller considered an operation essential and decided to try chloroform. Three students were hastily sent out of the hospital in search of Simpson, but he did not keep an appointment book and could not be found. Miller could wait no longer and proceeded to operate without any anaesthetic at all. He had only made his first cut when the patient fainted. He never recovered consciousness and died with the operation unfinished. Had chloroform had been used and the patient died, its whole career, as Simpson said to himself, "would have been arrested". Operations were few and far between, but on Friday 10 November, Simpson came over to the Infirmary and asked Miller if any surgery was to be carried out that day. It so happened that there were to be three operations, two by Miller and one by Dr John Duncan. Miller's first was on a child of six with an injured and now decaying bone in his arm. Simpson and Miller agreed to try the new drug.

Word got around, and the theatre was even more crowded than usual, and the child screamed and struggled as he was carried into the midst of the terrifying scene. His family came from the West and he only spoke Gaelic and no one had explained to him why his arm hurt, why he was here, or what awful thing was going to happen. He kicked and fought even more as everyone waited while Simpson took a bottle out of his pocket and poured the chloroform on to his own handkerchief. He approached the squirming child and tried to hold it over his face. The boy resisted, but was gently restrained by Simpson who made him breathe the sickly sweet fumes. In a few moments he relaxed, snoring away in a deep sleep.

Miller's operation notes state that "after a few inspirations the boy ceased to cry or move. A deep incision was now made down to the diseased bone and by the use of forceps nearly the whole of the radius in the state of sequestrum was extracted. During this operation and the subsequent examination of the wound by the finger, not the slightest evidence of the suffering of pain was given. He still slept soundly and was carried away to his ward in that state. Half an hour afterwards he was found in bed like a child newly awakened from a refreshing sleep, with a clear merry eye and placid expression of countenance, wholly unlike what is found to obtain after ordinary etherisation. On being questioned by a Gaelic interpreter who was found among the students he stated that he never felt any pain and that he felt none now. On being shown his wounded arm he looked much surprised, but neither cried nor otherwise expressed the slightest alarm."

Miller's other patient was a soldier, needing a very painful operation on the face. This time Simpson soaked a sponge in chloroform, rather than re-use his handkerchief. The operation was carried out and the soldier, emerged from his sweet chloro-formed dreams he showed his appreciation by grabbing the impregnated sponge and shoving it back over his mouth hoping to prolong his ecstasy rather than come back to reality! Dr John Duncan's patient was equally oblivious to the amputation of his very sensitive toe.

Quite by chance, among the throne watching the operations, was a visitor from France, Professor Dumas, Dean of the Faculty of Science in Paris—the first chemist to ascertain and establish the chemical composition of chloroform. He was delighted to be present, and Simpson the quick to point out the connection between the visitor and the drug being demonstrated that day.

Simpson now added a postscript to his pamphlet on the use of the new anaesthetic in midwifery, with a description of its successful use in the wider field of surgery. He also states that he had already exhibited chloroform on more than 50 occasions. The pamphlet, with these additional notes was published on 15 November, and 4,000 copies were sold within a few days, with many thousands more afterwards. Simpson had dedicated it to Professor Dumas and it bore the words of Bacon "I esteem it the office of a physician not only to restore health, but to mitigate pain and doctors".

The lay as well as the medical press now began to be full of

accounts of the use of chloroform, and Simpson's mail overflowed with letters from the public as well as doctors,
eulogising the magical fumes of what was now considered "his"
drug. The tremendous acclaim came because, to the people of
Edinburgh at least, Simpson had stopped *their* pain. It did not
matter to them that someone in the U.S.A. had done so already,
or that chemists had been scrutinising their test tubes for years.
A typical letter from the vast corresopndence of 1847 is from the
Duchess of Argyll.

> Rosneath, November 27th.
>
> Dear Dr Simpson
>
> I cannot resist writing one line to wish you joy of your dis-
> covery. I think your life must be a very happy one from the
> reliefs of *not* witnessing pain which must be as painful to see
> as to bear . . . I think you *should* have warned Mrs Simpson
> before you tried the chloroform! The Duke joins me in
> congratulating you.
>
> E. Argyll.

Liston wrote enthusiastically from London that he much
preferred chloroform to ether, and was now using it constantly;
and local papers carried reports of the use of chloroform
throughout the country. The *Carlisle Post* described the extraction of a tooth from an itinerant Irishman.

> The tooth was examined and he was desired to seat him-
> self in a chair, when a few drops of chloroform sprinkled on a
> handkerchief were held before his face; in a few seconds he
> began to fumble in his waistcoat pocket, from which he with-
> drew a short pipe and some tobacco, and requested that the
> lady (a nurse) might fetch him a light; by this time the effect
> of vapour had ceased, and he apologised for the liberty he
> had taken, which he considered was "all owing to that beau-
> tiful perfume". The quantity of chloroform given had not
> been sufficient to produce a state of unconsciousness. A larger
> quantity was now sprinkled on the handkerchief which was
> again held before his face, and in less than a minute he was
> sound asleep, the tooth was extracted, and he continued
> snoring for a minute longer, when he began to show symp-

toms of waking, and the following dialogue ensued:—"How are you now? where have you been?" "Well, I'll tell you, I was at Carlisle, and I went to the Infirmary there, and at first I sat down in a room with a lot of people, and then a gentleman whom I had never seen before called me out and asked me what I wanted, and I told him that I wanted to have an axle tooth taken out, for it had been troubling me long, and he told me to sit down in a chair, and I did, and then I breathed a beautiful perfume, and then. . . ." "Well, what then?" "Why then I went to that world that sinful mortals on earth often think about," and here he paused as if considering, and then suddenly exclaimed, "I think I am that same old sinner that went to the Infirmary myself", and again paused to consider, "but if it's the same I've got a loose axle tooth in my head". "Then you'd better feel if you have". The Irishman did as he was desired and carefully examined his jaw, and having apparently convinced himself said "No, there is no axle tooth, then I'm not the same". The effect of the vapour now rapidly subsided, and he speedily came to the conclusion that he was the same person, and that there must have been magic, and left the room evidently well satisfied at having so agreeably got rid of his troublesome companion.

Chloroform could do anything! An account was published in the *Bristol Mirror* of a cure of typhus fever: a girl of eighteen was kept in a sleepy chloroformed state for several days, twenty-four minims inhaled over forty minutes every four hours, with beef tea, porter and wine to keep her going, after which she recovered completely. Another paper reported that on a domestic use of chloroform: "A few nights ago a party of gentlemen tarried over their cups to an unreasonably late hour, and one of the number expressed some apprehension of a 'certain lecture'. A wag present suggested the use of chloroform, and accordingly the handkerchiefs of the party were duly sprinkled." When the wives' tirade began, the handkerchiefs were waved, and the ladies sent into a gentle oblivious sleep. The *North British Mail* described a case where not only the patient but the surgeon too had fallen into a deep sleep for fully ten minutes. The *John O'Groat Journal* reported:

Chloroform in Kirkwall—The new agent for preventing pain in surgical operations etc., was successfully employed on the 11th ult., by Dr James S. S. Logie of Kirkwall, who assisted by Dr Duguid, also of that place, removed a large tumour from the arm of a patient while under its influence. During the performance of the operation the patient was altogether unconscious of what was going on, and appeared rather to be in a state of happy delirium than in that of a sleep. He laughed and spoke frequently, as if to his wife and one of his neighbours, supposing them to be present, though neither of them was within twenty miles of him. In about a quarter of an hour after the operation had been finished he recovered from his delirium, but had no idea that the operation had been performed until the tumour was shown to him, upon which he expressed great surprise as well as joy. It had been growing for a period of 12 years, and was found to weigh, after its removal 1 lb to 7 oz. This is the first application of Professor Simpson's new anaesthetic agent in Orkney.

News travelled remarkably quickly, and before the end of November, chloroform apparently was readily available throughout the land, even, apparently, off the West Coast of Scotland. The local paper reported:

Narrow Escape—Application for Chloroform.
On the morning of Friday week, a Rothesay horse dealer proceeded to the quay with a horse for shipment to Glasgow. On reaching the quay, the horse most pertinaciously refused to leave terra firma. His master, however, determined to force the animal into the boat, and in a struggle which ensued, the gangway was pushed over the quay, and the stubborn horse, with its resolute master, were precipitated into the water. Undutiful though his steed had been on land, it did not forsake him in so ungenial an element. The man was ultimately rescued from his perilous position, and removed home, when it was found that his shoulder was dislocated. Drs McLauchlan and McEwan were speedily in attendance but it was found impossible, from the cries and resistance of the patient, to replace the bones. In these

circumstances, the medical gentlemen had recourse to the application of chloroform, which took immediate effect. The obstreperous patient became not only pliant, but also so elevated, that he commenced singing and bargaining about horses. On his restoration to consciousness, he was astonished to learn that all had been put to rights, whilst he had not experienced the slightest pain. The horse, on its owner being taken out of the water, swam to the east shore, where it was speedily rescued, without having been at all injured.— *Renfrewshire Advertiser.*

Not only vets, but butchers too began to reach for the bottle of chloroform. Christmas is a fatal period for pigs, and a Mr Horace Watson of the village of Laceby near Grimsby found it easier to use than a hammer. The animals were bled, scalded, cut up and salted "apparently not a bit the wiser for what had passed".

One, however, unsuspected difficulty was jumped on by the press, as it would today:

Science Impeded by the Excise—we understand that the distinguished discoverer of the effects of chloroform, to obviate the difficulty experienced by his brethren of the faculty in London in procuring the article in a state of purity, lately essayed to forward a small quantity from the laboratory of Messrs Duncan and Flockhart, of this town when lo! it was seized by the excise upon the border. Chloroform of course, does not contain one particle of spirit, but it is quite possible that spirit is employed in its preparation, although it is just as possible, we believe, to prepare it without. This little incident is like to show us that we have hardly yet got beyond the verge of the times when Galileo's astronomy was forced to bow to the dogmas of the Inquisition. It is quite wonderful what the vigilance of excisemen will prompt them sometimes to seize. We have heard of a late instance on the border of the seizure of coffee, and all because a few drops of spirits had been used as a preservative. This, however, might be the means of saving the conscientious scruples of a pledged teatotaller.—*North British Mail.*

By September 1848 chloroform had reached the outposts of the Empire. Corporal Ryder of the 32nd Foot wrote home while fighting with the army in India near Mooltan that he had seen a man's leg amputated "under the operation of chloroform. He never stirred the least under the operation and knew nothing of what was going on . . .he felt nothing nor did he know it was off until he looked!"

Some public opinion, however, now took on a different shade. As Simpson remarked, it was only when a means of preventing pain had been established that arguments were produced against its use.

Anaesthesia was unnatural. According to various doctors particularly Meigs of Philadelphia, it was quite unnecessary. How could a mother love her child if she did not suffer for it? After all, pain was of moral value, to be borne unflinchingly.

A Liverpool doctor, another Petrie, considered anaesthesia a breach of medical ethics. It was the act of a coward, he wrote, to avoid pain, and if a woman insisted on the use of chloroform to alleviate her labour pains, she must be told that she was in no fit state to make decisions. "Are we going to allow the patient to tell us what to do?" he enquired indignantly. Others, men and women safely past childbearing years quoted their Bible: "In sorrow thou shalt bring forth children" (Gen. 3:16). Pain, they said, was a part of God's purpose, and the curse after the fall. The controversy had been preceded in the same year 1847, by an article in which Professor Miller described anaesthesia. Dr Chalmers, the Free Church leader, who had been present at operations under anaesthetic, had been invited to contribute a theological section to Miller's article, but had refused on the grounds that there were no theological issues, whatever "small theologians" might say. Miller's article appeared in the *North British Review* for May 1847, alongside articles on the sanitary condition of the labouring population, and on Madagascar, especially as a missionary field. It began with some apology for introducing a matter which "yet touches all members of the human family alike; or if there be any difference, patients are more interested than practitioners—the laity more than the profession—the mass more than the medical section of mankind. . . . Even editors and critics must stoop to arrange themselves among the benefitted; and in this question may well say—

confessing their humanity and throwing aside for once the almost superhuman obscurity in which they have to dwell— *Homo sum, humani nihil a me alienum puto.*"

Simpson's character was exactly built to cope with arguments such as these, and he assumed full responsibility for placing his chloroform above suspicion, and to make good his claim to its merits. His crusade in particular was to make chloroform available to every woman in labour. There was no alternative to their anguish. Prophylaxis and Grantly Dick Reid, when their time came, were a far cry from Simpson's times with the Victorian woman writhing in her Industrial Revolution slum, or squashed into an overcrowded Lying-in-Hospital with a pelvis distorted from malnutrition, or the more refined ladies, terrified that this confinement could be as frightful as their last.

Simpson resolved to beat down all opposition, particularly that of the pious and sanctimonious men of his profession. Someone else could and would have discovered the anaesthetic properties of chloroform, but it needed a Simpson to make the doing part of every doctor's armamentarium and to make it every woman's right to be able to receive it. Characteristically, Simpson tackled the most formidable opposition first, that of the medical profession. The charge levelled against chloroform was that it would increase the already high death rate following operations. With common sense Simpson saw that the only method of finding the truth was by collecting a vast number of statistics comparing the results of operations with and without the use of an anaesthetic. Simpson wrote to every hospital in the country for their returns and also to Paris; he then scrutinised their reports. Amputation of the thigh was the operation most dreaded by surgeons, two out of three patients dying as a result. Simpson's figures showed that out of 145 anaesthetised patients, only 37 died, or one in three.

His very long and detailed paper on this subject appeared in the Edinburgh Monthly Journal of Medical Science in April 1848. It was headed with two quotations:

"Why dost thou whet thy knife so earnestly?"
"Shylock must be merciful".
"On what compulsion must I? Tell me that." (*The Merchant of Venice*).

In summing up Simpson pointed out that an anaesthetic saves the patient from pain; and a good proportion of people from death as well, by avoiding the physical and mental shock of the operation and its consequences.

The medical profession countered with a suggestion from Dublin that the use of chloroform in childbirth would increase the incidence of bleeding, paralysis, pneumonia, and so on. Simpson immediately collected statistics from the Dublin hospitals, and flourished them in the face of his critics. He proved then, and again afterwards, the pain itself and the shock and exhaustion it caused were far greater dangers than any resulting from the use of an anaesthetic.

Simpson answered the serious objection that chloroform brought on mania in the mother by visiting the Edinburgh lunatic asylum. Eleven patients were confined there with puerperal mania, but not one had had chloroform administered during her delivery.

Charles Meigs, of Philadelphia was not the only one who considered the pain of labour beneficial. An Edinburgh doctor wrote in the *Medical and Surgical Journal* of July 1847: "In the lying in chamber, pain is the mother's safety, its absence her destruction." They were not referring to natural labours, but to those in which instruments were considered necessary. Answering a letter from Simpson Meigs asked how he could be sure he adjusted the forceps blade accurately except by asking the patient if it hurt?

The critics on religious issues were dealt with on their own ground by quotations from the Bible. It is interesting to note that the loudest and most persistent objections came not from the church, but from members of Simpson's own profession. The church leaders, such as Dr Chalmers, saw no objection. The reply to the much quoted verse—"In sorrow thou shalt bring forth children"—was that the Hebrew word "Etzebh" did not mean suffering in the sense of pain, but was better rendered as "labour, toil or physical exertion". Simpson reiterated the point that on the occasion of the first recorded operation—the removal of a rib—the Lord had caused a deep sleep to fall on Adam, proof of his approval of anaesthesia!

A Dr Samuel Ashwell took up this point in the *Lancet*. "Dr Simpson surely forgets that the deep sleep of Adam took place

before the introduction of pain into the world during his state
of Innocence." Simpson replied vigorously,

> I will not offend you by comparing the theological opinion of
> John Calvin with that of Samuel Ashwell, but let me ask you
> one single question, is it anywhere stated in your Bible that
> pain came in with sin, or that there was no pain endured
> when there was no sin? If so, then let me add, your Bible
> differs from mine . . . If you refuse to interfere with a natural
> function because it is natural, why do you ride my dear
> doctor? You ought to talk, in order to be consistent. Chloro-
> form does nothing but save pain, you allege. A carriage does
> nothing but save fatigue. Which is more important to be done
> away with? Your fatigue or your patients' screams and tor-
> tures?"

Simpson also enquired if Dr Ashwell wore clothes. Most
unnatural if he did!

Simpson gathered together his answers to criticism and
published them in the most famous of all his pamphlets,
"Answer to the Religious Objections Advanced Against the
Employment of Anaesthetic Agents in Midwifery and Surgery".
This was headed by two telling New Testament texts: "For
every creature of God is good and nothing to be refused, if it be
received with thanksgiving" (Tim. 4:4); "Therefore to him
that knoweth to do good and doeth it not, to him it is sin"
(Jas. 4:17).

The pamphlet argued that Christ's mission was to introduce
mercy, not sacrifice. Also, it reminded those who held blindly
to the law written in Genesis that thistles and thorns which the
land grows should never be uprooted and no one should eat with
a merry heart of food not earned by their own physical labour.
From time immemorial opiates, instruments, laxatives and
stimulants had been resorted to to allieviate the pain of childbirth, and no one's conscience had been disturbed in the matter
before. Only now that the sufferings of the mother could be
relieved entirely, had the objections bestirred themselves to
complain.

Simpson also pointed out that the black woman was cured

by God as well as the white, yet some of the black tribes of the human race suffer little physical pain during parturition; surely it could not be considered irreligious to reduce the physical sufferings of the civilised sister?

Simpson's final thrust to his critics was to remind them that many clergymen still considered it a heinous crime to vaccinate against smallpox although during the fifty years since its introduction, the number of lives saved by the vaccination equalled the entire population of Wales! "Some went so far as to pronounce innoculation an invention of Satan himself, because it interfered with the intentions of God."

Simpson's paper silenced those who objected on religious grounds, but it is interesting to note that in 1957 Pope Pius XII still found it necessary to reiterate Simpson's arguments. In his "Address in Reply to 3 Questions Concerning Religious and Moral Aspects of Pain Prevention in Medical Practice" his Holiness stated: ". . . Man even after the fall retains the right of control over the forces of nature . . . and consequently of deriving benefit from all the resources offered him to suppress or to avoid physical pain."

The opponents of the use of chloroform seemed to have already forgotten the horrors of the infliction of physical pain. Professor Miller gave support to his neighbour's battle by publicly recalling the days when a patient in a panic of fear was removed from the ward, yelling and sobbing, and attempting to escape the hefty assistants trying to hold him down as they hauled him to the operating theatre. One who did remember these times was a Dr George Wilson and his letter to Simpson surely settles any argument as to the right of a doctor to withhold an anaesthetic on any grounds whatsoever.

My dear Dr Simpson,
    I have recently read with mingled sadness and surprise the declarations of some surgeons that anaesthetics are needless luxuries and that unendurable agony is the best of tonics. Those surgeons, I think, can scarcely have been patients of their brother surgeons, and jest of scars only because they never felt a wound, but if they remain enemies of anaesthesia after what you have written I despair of convincing them of their utility.

Several years ago I was required to prepare on very short warning for the loss of a limb by amputation. A painful disease . . . suddenly became aggravated, and I was informed by two surgeons of the highest skill that I must choose between death and the sacrifice of the limb, and that the choice must be promptly made for my strength was sinking, under pain, sleeplessness and exhaustion.

The operation was a more tedious one than some which involve much greater mutilation. It necessitated cruel cutting through inflamed and morbidly sensitive parts and could not be despatched by a few swift strokes of the knife. . . . Of the agony it occasioned I will say nothing. Suffering so great as I underwent cannot be expressed in words and thus fortunately cannot be recalled. The particular pangs are now forgotten but the black whirlwind of emotion, the horror of great darkness and the sense of desertion by God and man bordering close on despair, which swept through my mind and overwhelmed my heart. I can never forget however gladly I would do so. Only the wish to save others some of my sufferings makes me deliberately recall and confess the anguish and humiliation of such a personal experience.

During the operation in spite of the pain it occasioned my senses were preternaturally acute as I have been told they generally are in patients in such circumstances. I watched all that the surgeon did with a fascinated intensity. I still recall with unwelcome vividness the spreading out of the instruments, the twisting of the tourniquet, the first incision, the fingering of the sawed bone, the spoon pressed on the flap, the tying of the blood vessels, the stitching of the skin and the bloody dismembered limb lying on the floor. These are not pleasant remembrances.

As for the fear entertained by some that the moral good which accrues from suffering, and is intended by the Ruler of All to be secured by it, will be lost if agony is evaded by sufferers having recourse to anaesthetics, we may surely leave that to the disposal of Him who does all things well. The best answer to such complaints I have heard was given by an excellent old lady to another who was doubting whether any of the daughters of Eve were at liberty to lessen by anaesthesia the pangs of child-bearing. "You need not be afraid", said the wiser lady, "that there will not be enough of suffering in the world."

Yours most truly,
An Old Patient.

Simpson's fighting attack systematically knocked down the objections of his opponents. He waged battle by endless letters, papers, pamphlets and lectures. He used chloroform extensively in his own practice, badgered others to do likewise, and he taught his students to do the same.

Among Simpson's class during this time was Francis De Quincey, who wrote to his father, Thomas, remarking on the "enthralling lectures of Simpson" and relating the series of ridiculous religious objections put forward by the medical profession. It was left to Simpson, who held the Chair of Midwifery, to teach the students the practice of anaesthetics. The only other professor who broached the subject was Syme, who dealt with it in one ten-minute lecture.

A study of Simpson's lectures on anaesthetics over the next twenty years as recorded by the student scribes demonstrates his continued search for insight into the subject. Every lecture refers to different letters received and new Continental and American books and papers read. The lectures delivered in 1862 are particularly revealing, and show his views on the subject now that his knowledge had been reinforced by experience. He first reminds the students that anything new meets with resistance. When the mail coach to London cut the time down from five to three nights and two days, the travellers were advised to rest at York, as several who had gone straight through were said to have died of apoplexy from the rapidity of the motion. As likely many of the deaths alleged to chloroform? Optical glasses, spectacles and the telescope were first spoken of by the church as "offsprings of man's wicked mind", because they changed the natural appearance of things and presented them in an untrue light. Tea and coffee were denounced by the Church when first introduced, as they had aphrodisiac properties, reminding Simpson of the case of the two old Edinburgh ladies who lived in the High Street and refused a present of some potatoes from their grocer, because they had heard of the aphrodisiac contained in the starch. Surprising that they should worry, Simpson pointed out, as they were well on into their seventies!

Fear of innovation is as deep in the military profession as in the medical. When it was proposed to abolish flogging, Simpson reminded the students, it was the officers who leapt to their feet in Parliament to oppose the bill, in the same way that the older accoucheur springs up in the ladies bedroom to oppose chloroform. The same horrible system of lashing is still practised in the Navy today, 1862, as in 1662. A Dr Marshall tells of a fellow being lately "lashed round the fleet" as a punishment for desertion. This meant thirty lashes in one ship, his raw bleeding flesh then wrapped in a blanket and handed over to the next ship, till three thousand lashes had been inflicted. This case of Dr Marshall's sank into exhaustion at the after two hundred and fifty lashes when he tsurgeon on board the ship anchored in the Firth of Forth, said he would not be answerable for his life. When the sailor had recovered, he was handed round the remaining ships, after which he died.

Simpson's sense of humour comes to the fore in these lectures to his students. He loved telling the story of how he silenced a Dr Parkes's objections to anaesthesia by enquiring if the piece of breakfast roll he had just swallowed caused him any pain. "'No,' he replied. 'Then you,' I said, 'are not fulfilling the curse which says in sorrow thou shalt eat of it all the days of your life.'" One objecting minister sent half of his congregation to sleep every time he delivered a sermon—"I wrote to him saying you must be as wicked a man as me."

Anaesthetics were blamed for everything, and Simpson would relate how "at the close of the twelfth century the mother of St Mungo of Glasgow, the grandson of a Pictish King, was confined to a monastery. She became, what nuns sometimes will—pregant. She pleaded innocence, denying any part in the act, alleging that it must have taken place while she was under a deep sleep, after partaking of the drink of oblivion—wine and madragora." Chloroform was blamed too for producing lewd lewd thoughts. If it does, warns Simpson, the doctor has only himself to blame, as the unconscious mind works on any conversation held directly before the induction! He quoted the case of a pretty young patient of Dr Dubois in Paris, who spoke kindly and lovingly during her operation to one of the students present. It turned out that she was his kept mistress! Surely, Simpson asked his intrigued audience, the anaesthetic was not at fault here? "Anaesthetics are accused too of producing idiocy in the child. One of the first champions of it was discussing the matter with Sir John Forbes, and mentioned Dr Graems objections, that is, that the child would be made "What a piece of impudence" Sir John replied "on the part of Simpson to assert that he was the first to use chloroform; why, it must have been given to Graems mother when she brought him into the world more than forty years ago!"

One of Simpson's class argued that some patients could not be anaesthetised—him for instance. That evening his fellow students forced him to inhale a handkerchief liberally sprinkled with chloroform, took his clothes off, put a baby's feeder round his neck, and rang for his landlady. The professor enjoyed the joke and told the story to every succeeding year of students.

Simpson goes very fully into the reports of deaths from chloroform. Most he dismisses as due to impurities in the drug, or faulty administration. In his three articles on the subject, and in his student lectures he points out very carefully that certain rules must be obeyed in order to produce a successful anaesthetic effect. First, the patient must be left quiet and calm during the induction and recovery; second, there should be a quick induction to avoid the primary state of excitement; and third, nothing must be done towards the operation until the patient is properly asleep. Struggling and choking are caused only by bad administration or impurities in the drug. Morton, the American, in his thesis on the administration of ether, stresses exactly the same points. The chloroform must be pure, reiterated Simpson again and again. The highest incidence of death from chloroform came from America. Dr Warren reported ten from the Massachusettes General Hospital during six months. Three of these were from operations connected with dentistry; two were induced by doctors with no previous experience, and the other patient had been under the influence of chloroform on several occasions before with no bad effect, but on this occasion died instantly. Simpson assessed the symptoms preceeding death, and declared that the patients had been poisoned by impure chloroform. He immediately wrote to Dr Meigs and sent off a bottle of his own drug, as produced by Duncan and Flockhart of Edinburgh. Dr Meigs refused the sample and was adamant that the U.S.A. could and did produce chloroform of an even higher standard than Edinburgh!

Most reports of death due to chloroform, Simpson stated, were not established. On one occasion the patient, a young boy suffering from a stone in his bladder had smothered under the impregnated cloth while the six doctors present argued about the site of the stone. They turned round to find the boy dead. A rag wet with water would give the same result! The antidote to chloroform was oxygen and Simpson urged that this should always be kept ready for emergency use. At this point in his lecture Simpson would read the following from *The Times*.

Tuesday, March 12th, 1850.

Prejudice against chloroform—We observe it stated that chloroform has been employed in Edinburgh, in from 80,000 to 100,000 cases, without a single accident or bad effect of any kind attributable to its use. Mr Carmichael, a surgeon of that city, commenting on the fact, says, "Would 80,000 or 100,000 full doses of opium, or antimony, or Epsom salts, or any other potent medicine, have been followed with as great impunity?" Chloroform is now habitually used in Edinburgh in all kinds of surgical operations, down to tooth drawing. It saves many lives which otherwise would sink under the nervous shock which is experienced from a severe operation undergone in a state of consciousness. Such is the published opinion of the discoverer of its use as an anaesthetic, the now celebrated Dr J. Y. Simpson; and this opinion has not been gainsaid by any of the profession in Edinburgh. At the same time chloroform has received the sanction and recommendation of the most authoritative bodies in France and the United States. Nevertheless, the public of London is almost wholly denied the vast benefit of this agent, purely through the prejudices of the profession. This forms a curious illustration of the medical mind in the metropolis, but it is not a new one. Not only is there a distaste amongst scientific men in England for everything that comes from the north, but there is a general benightedness in the London medical world. They opposed vaccination while it was embraced in the provinces; and to the indelible disgrace of all concerned, inoculation with small pox maintained its ground in a London hospital devoted to the purpose a quarter of a century after Jenner's discovery. The London public should take this matter into their own hands.

If chloroform did produce one death from poor administration, Simpson asked his class, was it right to give it up? Every medicine listed in the Pharmacopoiea then in use should be scrapped in such a case. According to the Registrar General, 242 deaths were recorded in 1844 as a result of poisons, all of which had been prescribed as medicinal!

Actually, Simpson was not entirely satisfied with chloroform himself, and he continued to research into other possibilities and also into the question of local anaesthetics. Each lecture to his students covered a wider field and included new and additional anecdotes. Every member of Simpson's household by now was haphazardly sniffing anything he produced. On one occasion he resolved to try the effect of a mixture of chloroform and aerated water and produced this at a dinner in his house. Hearing of this, his butler removed what was left and gave it to the cook, saying it was champagne. She gulpted it down and promptly fell insensible on to the kitchen floor. The butler rushed upstairs calling for Simpson, shouting, "I've poisoned the cook. For God's sake come down." Fortunately she recovered.

Simpson related an incident concerning himself and a lady patient: "I remember one morning inhaling some carbonated hydrogen, and eight hours later I was called out. The lady I attended remarked very gravely that she thought gas must be escaping somewhere. I never, of course let on though perfectly well aware where the gas escaped!"

Simpson described to his students his numerous experiments on earthworms, leeches and guinea pigs' legs in a search for a local anaesthetic so far he had met with no success on humans. He involved his students with his line of thought, expecting them to think, rather than just swallow facts as was the practice. He asked them, for instance, why in the earthworm, "If the nervous system were affected through the circulation, the animal's rings should be paralysed longitudinally in the direction of the connecting ganglia, as well as transversely, which they are not." On this question, Simpson related that "My friend Dr Adams had his lower extremities immersed in liquid chloroform for more than half a day, at the end of which period he thought they were completely anaesthetised, firmly believing that chloroform could produce local anaesthesia. I then sent an electric shock through one of his legs, at which he gave a most unanaesthetic roar and yell!"

Simpson considered freezing to be the best local anaesthetic, but it was troublesome and expensive. His friend Dr Andrews had invented a machine to use solid carbonic acid, at a most of three shillings per application, but "I think it will explode". Simpson was sceptical about the use of "galvanism", or the administration of an electric shock, to produce local anaesthesia. Dentists for a long time were partial to this measure. "The patient after having his tooth seized by the dental forceps had an electric shock passed through the nerve of the tooth, while at the same time the dentist gave a good wrench and pulled it out. These two operations were followed by an unearthly yell from the patient who was hastily assured that the pain came from the electricity used, and not the pulling of the tooth—just like the boy at school offering to pull out a hair painlessly. This he does by giving the other lad such a whack on the side of the head, that this alone is felt." At present, Simpson declared, there was nothing to offer the patient sufficiently numbing to enable him to stand the knife or cautery. Chloroform mixed with belladona was the strongest so far, and this Simpson used in the form of pills, as we would aspirin today.

The series of lectures on anaesthesia ended with the following statement: "With all this furore for and against chloroform, the main point seems to be completely overlooked; that of the views of the patient. I mean, the complete immunity from pain which the patient experiences when placed under the influence of the drug." Nothing terrifies man more than the surgeon's knife. "Mr Liston used to tell the story of Lord Dundonald, the most brave seaman, when while fearlessly boarding the *Esmeralda* was knocked down by a Spanish sailor and fell back into his own boat, hitting his thigh on a thole pin. Liston went several times to remove the resulting tumour, but the brave and dauntless admiral always lost courage at the sight of the knife and delayed the operation from day to day."

Simpson continually urged careful use of the new drug, and pointed out its potential dangers to his students, and to doctors in letters sent far and wide.

Nevertheless, reports of death did appear and with alarming frequency. The earlier anaesthetic ether had also cast its toll, the first death recorded by the *Lancet* in 27 March, 1847, was of Ann Parkinson who was operated on on 9 March for the removal of a tumour of her thigh. She never rallied, and died forty hours later on 11 March. She was twenty-one, the wife of a hairdresser of Spittlegate, near Grantham, who had been married one and a half years and had a child of nine months. During the previous year a tumour, that had grown on the under part of her left thigh, became so large it "became a perpetual torment to her, as she was unable to sit or lie down in bed". On her death, the coroner was called in, an inquiry instigated, and the doctor faced with a charge of criminal negligence, inattention or rashness, which would lead to a verdict of manslaughter. The jury came to the conclusion. however, that the entire fault lay in the ether, and the doctor was let off with an admonition.

The *Lancet*'s first recording of death from chloroform was 5 February 1848 when Hannah Greene died after the administration of chloroform for the excision of the nail of her big toe. Hannah was fifteen, said to be strong, apart from her diseased feet. When she failed to rally after the operation, the doctor had dashed water in her face and put brandy in her mouth, but the brandy rattled in her throat. He bled her in the arm and neck, but very little flowed. She never recovered. At the post mortem the lungs were said to be full of bloody froth and the epiglottis of a vermilion hue. The mucous membrane of the larynx was redder than usual, mottled with vascular petechiae. The stomach was distended with food. The inquest recorded death from congestion of the lungs, due to the inhalation of chloroform. Simpson was up in arms at this finding: he maintained that Hannah Greene had in fact drowned from having brandy poured into her mouth when unconscious. The next issues of the *Lancet* carried rude and scathing letters of opposition, and equally devastating accusations and replies.

Simpson himself records no deaths from chloroform until 1870.

On February 5th, I chloroformed a patient with a single layer of towel over the nose and mouth, leaving the eyes exposed. When Mr Brotherstone of Alloa made the first cutaneous incision, the patient moved so much that he stopped for a brief time till I put the patient more deeply under the effects of anaesthetic. Mr Brotherstone was introducing his hand with the view to turning out the ovarian mass when the patient vomited suddenly and profusely. Immediately the eyes opened; the pupils were preternaturally dilated. The face looked pallid; and the respiration which had never been affected by the chloroform so as to have the least noise or stertor in it, seemed arrested. Instantly artificial respiration was set on foot, and the tongue pulled forward. Deep spontaneous respiration then occured and I deemed at the moment that the patient was out of danger but a second collapse occurred, which terminated in death, all means of resuscitation proving unavailing.

It has been stated that Simpson supressed other cases where chloroform was considered the cause of death, such as that of the thin, delicate Mrs H. who went to Dr Roberts in 1855 in Edinburgh for the extraction of three teeth. She collapsed, and the dentist sent his son immediately round the corner to contact Simpson, who came at once. All methods of resuscitation were tried including galvanism but with no success. This was Dr Roberts' 2,097th chloroform case. In Simpson's notes to his students, he records this case in detail, and puts the death down to the excited state of the patient who had died of fear, not chloroform. Attributing the death to the nervous state of the patient may not be wishful thinking on his part: the danger of chloroform is now known to be fibrillation—uncoordinated beating—of the heart, a condition greatly aggravated by the excess adrenalin found in the apprenhensive patient. Simpson constantly reminded people to calm the patient, keep the instruments out of sight, and not to discuss the operation. His benevolent expression, striking appearance and genuine hummanity must have had a profound effect in preventing this fatal complication. Of course if she had not relied on the anaesthetic, she would never have faced having the teeth out and so might have lived a full span.

Joseph Lister recorded that in 1861 Syme, now the leading surgeon in Scotland, had performed 5,000 operations under chloroform, and had never lost a patient through its use. It is therefore no wonder that Duncan and Flockhart, the Edinburgh chemists, were doing a flourishing trade. In fact their name became synonymous with chloroform in many parts of the world. Mr Duncan had founded the shop in 1820 in the new buildings on the North Bridge. Flockhart joined the partnership later. He was a surgeon as well as a druggist, and a man of boundless energy. It is said that when the closing hour of the shop was changed from 11.00 to 9.00 p.m. he was ashamed to go home so early! His familiar tall figure was seen at every gathering and function in Edinburgh, and he was involved in every public affair and issue of the times. Duncan preferred to potter about in his herb garden, just outside the city beyond Liberton, but would come up to the shop every day on his pony, which he stabled at the York Hotel, opposite the Royal College of Surgeons. Both men were part of the medical circle in Edinburgh, and had many friends among the University Medical Faculty and the practising doctors of the town. They were always ready to make up any medicinal concoction, and the result was always of the highest standard. It was natural for Simpson to have turned to this partnership for a sample of chloroform when Waldie had failed to send him some from Liverpool.

After 4 November 1847, 52 North Bridge was a hive of activity, replenishing supplies of chloroform. The early methods of preparing chloroform were often dangerous. On one occasion a retort exploded, but luckily the two chemists had their spectacles on. The quality of their product must have been particularly good, as, in 1926, some of their earliest chloroform was tested, and was found to be little different from the finest made now. The bleaching-powder method they used was popular up to 1946. By 1855 the firm was making 7,000 doses a day and by 1870 this had been stepped up to 8,000.

Duncan and Flockhart's chloroform went round the world, speeded on its way by the Grindlay family shipping interests. The *Betsy* and the *Orpheus* carried the drug to Jamaica and Bahia where it was sold at 4/– an ounce, a profit of 1/–! Simpson had money invested in both these ships, but there is no record of how much the family made on this transaction!

The arguments for and against the use of chloroform continued until 1853 when it became known that the indomitable Queen Victoria herself had taken chloroform from the hands of a Dr John Snow, during the birth of Prince Leopold, on 7 April 1853. The Queen was most enthusiastic about its use, and she knew what she was talking about too, for this was her eighth confinement.

Her Majesty's physician, Dr J. Clark, immediately informed Simpson of the successful result. It has been suggested that the great decision to allow the thirty-four-year-old Queen the benefit of chloroform was actually made by Albert. The Queen's doctors were reluctant to assume the responsibility, but when forced to it, they hastily called in Dr Snow. He was even more aware of the dangers of chloroform than they were, and, in fact, was collecting material for a paper reviewing the deaths from the drug during the first ten years. This was published after his own death, and dealt with fifty, twenty-five in England, six in Scotland and ninetten from the rest of the world.

Since 1847 John Snow had been intrigued with the idea of unconsciousness, and had limited his medical practice to anaesthetics; he was the son of a Yorkshire farmer, and, as an apprentice doctor, he had been involved in the cholera outbreak in Newcastle in 1832. He was in London when the use of, first ether, then chloroform came to light, and immediately became interested in the question of anaesthetics. He had already published a paper on the "Asphyxia and Resusitation of the New Born Child", and this subject was just his life. He was quiet and retiring, and enjoyed the transformation in the operating theatre since the use of anaesthesia. He had worked with Liston, and although he considered ether safer than chloroform, he much preferred to use the latter. He devised various types of inhalers, disapproving strongly of Simpson's happy-go-lucky method of dripping the drug onto a handkerchief. Snow was particularly horrified when he heard of one occasion during a confinement when the chloroform bottle had been knocked over, and spilled on the carpet. Without a murmur Simpson had got out his penknife, cut a piece off the carpet and held it in front of the patient who inhaled, and slept on regardless. By the use of Snow's machine, an accurate dose could be ascertained, and it was his portable inhaler that he carried to the Palace on the spring evening of 7 April. According to his diary, however, he used Simpson's handkerchief method, after all; sprinkling the chloroform on to it and the Queen inhaled for fifty-three minutes, expressing "herself greatly relieved by the administration". The court circular was silent on the subject, and Snow's name was never mentioned among the attending doctors Presumably they were ashamed of having given in to the Queen —although everyone knew that it was nearly impossible to refuse her once her mind had been made up! The *Lancet* actually denied the fact that chloroform was used, but the lay press, and the *Associated Medical Journal* (later to become the *British Medical Journal*) jumped on the news. Simpson made no secret of his letter from Dr Clark, and soon everyone was talking of the event. The Queen and her infant son seemed to be making a very quick recovery; particularly significant since she had already caused a stir by insisting on getting dressed and appearing in public a few days after her previous confinements instead of staying in the usual three-week purdah.

All the doctors in the country must have winced, knowing that now every woman would be demanding chloroform, and that their thin excuses for refusing it had gone for ever. The sensible Queen would never have taken it, their patients would say, if there really was any substance in the objection that it was dangerous, or against the will of the Lord. The country knew, too, that the hypochondriac Prince Albert would have weighed up the pros and cons with his usual German thoroughness before raising the subject with Dr Clark. Clark was a Scot, who qualified at Aberdeen, then practised as a naval surgeon. He attended Keats in Rome and had been appointed by Prince Leopold who then recommended him to Victoria's mother in 1835. He had a mania for fresh air and had published a thesis on the subject. He had a theory on "air conditioning" and wanted to install a blower into Buckingham Palace but was scoffed at by the Queen. He practised Gregorian physic—along with rhubarb and ipecacuana pills. He had caused a furore in court circles by suggesting that a lady in waiting, Flora Hastings, was pregant when the poor young girl was desperately ill and dying of a liver tumour. He is accused, too, of mismanaging the typhoid that killed Prince Albert. However, he was prepared to call in Snow to administer chloroform to Victoria and thereby set the seal for the drug's success.

Four years later, when the scene at the Palace was re-enacted for the birth of Princess Beatrice, the climate of opinion had changed: even the *Lancet* carried the news, and Snow's name was officially included among those in the Queen's room.

This was not the first time that Victoria had set an example to the country: as a child, she had been the first member of the Royal Family to be vaccinated for smallpox.

By 1853 anaesthetic practice had assumed certain distinctive characteristics in different parts of the world. In the northern States of America ether was used; the southern States traditionally followed the example of Paris in medical matters, and in Paris chloroform was administered from a handkerchief, according to Simpson's directions. The rest of Europe also followed Parisian methods, and in Scotland, of course, Simpson's method reigned supreme. In England a very different state of affairs obtained. Because of John Snow's strong influence, the English from the first considered the giving of an anaesthetic to be a specialist's job (elsewhere the task of administration was usually relegated to a junior or relation of the patient). By the beginning of 1848 the English had already devised a number of chloroform inhalers, and Snow was controlling the anaesthetic mixture by regulating the temperature in the vaporising chamber by means of a water jacket. Snow's portable regulating chloroform inhaler served his contemporaries as a model until the introduction of Clover's chloroform apparatus in 1862. After Snow's death in 1858, Clover had quietly become recognised as the leader in anaesthetic practice, and it was chiefly through his influence that a committee of investigation of the Royal Medical and Chirurgical Society in 1877 was formed to carry out experiments on ether and chloroform. It came to the conclusion that no single agent could be expected completely to satisfy every requirement and that there was a place for both.

In 1935 the British College of Obstetrics and Gynaecology was still at the subject, and organised an investigation into the use of an anaesthetic that could be administered by midwives. It concluded that chloroform was unsuitable, as, out of 4,577 patients considered, 6 had died. However in 1947 a survey was carried out and it was found that 94 per cent of the general practitioners in Britain used chloroform in their practice. In January 1950 the *British Medical Journal* carried a letter from a doctor who had "administered the drug on 3,319 separate occasions with 1 death. . . . To favour chloroform in labour may class one among the diehards, but I still remain faithful . . .".

Now chloroform has officially fallen into disrepute, but it is significant that a highly thought-of Edinburgh obstetrician when questioned by the author admitted to "giving a wee whiff of chloroform" to this very day; and a recent textbook selected at random from the library shelves gives details of the technique used to employ it.

Chloroform has therefore lost its place in the dental chair and operating theatre, to linger on its original domain, the room of the woman in labour. Be that as it may, in 1895 *The Times* carried a review of the numerous delicate operations that had come into practice in the latter half of the century, the paper remarks, "But where should we have been without anaesthetics? No human being could undergo in a conscious state such operations as we have spoken of. We doubt if anyone could nerve himself to perform them. We place the name of Simpson at the head of the list for true credit. He fought the fight of anaesthesia."

CHAPTER IX

Prime

SIMPSON WAS NOW in his prime. But his work on chloroform was only one amongst many incidents in a busy life, and the years 1847 and '48 left him and his way of life unchanged. His mind was now occupied with another problem: infection. In March 1848 he read a paper to the Edinburgh Medical Chirurgical Society on "Solutions of Gun Cotton, Gutta Percha and Caoutchouc as dressings for wounds". In December 1848 a further paper came out "The Contagiousness of Cholera". He had first written on this subject in 1838, when he considered the waves of cholera that regularly swept across Europe. Simpson then endorsed the theory that there was a direct infection from one patient to the next, an idea scoffed at by most British doctors because they did not believe in something they could not see. Now, in 1848, Simpson was beginning to wonder if the spread of infection and fevers from person to person was inevitable. Medical men were also asking why so many women died from a fever a few days after the difficulties of delivery were behind them; and Simpson was among the first to tie up the two problems and consider puerperal and surgical fever as one and the same. In the report for the Lying-in Hospital that Simpson submitted in this year, he wrote, "I have often stated and taught that if our present medical, surgical and obstetric hospitals were changed from being crowded places—a layer of sick in each flat—into villages or cottages with . . . at most two patients in each room, a great saving of human life would be effected." The Edinburgh Lying-in Hospital had been recently moved from St John Street to the Canongate, but Simpson's far-sighted ideas were not put into effect in the new building—in fact he had not even appreciated why his system would have prevented the spread of infection and disease. The previous year Ignaz Semmelweis reported that he had greatly reduced the incidence of puerperal fever in his hospital in Vienna by insisting that all the attendants washed their hands in chlorinated water. Simpson was not greatly impressed with Semmelweis's theory, and only came back to the subject many years later. Meanwhile, he hurried about his daily life in Edinburgh.

The *Bombay Courier* of 22 January 1848 carried a letter from a doctor in the Indian Army who had just spent a leave in Europe. In this letter the doctor states that the most outstanding character that he had come across in his tour of the medical centres of Europe was "little Simpson of Edinburgh" who had, he considered, the four ideals for the perfect physician:

The brain of an Apollo, the eye of an eagle, the heart of a lion, and the hand of a lady—nothing baffles his intellect, nothing escapes his penetrating glance, he sticks at nothing and he bungles nothing. If his practice was worth a rupee per annum it is worth £10,000! [Twice as much as the Great Deliverer of Scotland ever realised!] . . . From all parts, not of Britain only, but Europe, do ladies rush to see, consult and fee the little man. He has spread joy throughout many a rich man's house by enabling his wife to present him with a living child—a feat that none but Simpson ever *dared* to enable her to do. To watch him of a morning with his poor patients (them only of course was I permitted to see) was a treat. In comes a woman with a fibrous tumour of the abdomen, which 50 other practitioners have called 50 other names. One minute suffices for his diagnosis; another sees her flung down on the bed in a state of insensibility and in less than a third, two long needles are thrust inches deep into the tumour and a galvanic battery is at work *discussing* it. Leave her alone quietly, says Simpson, she'll take care of herself— no fear. What other men would speculate as to the propriety of for hours, Simpson *does* in a minute or two. He is bold but not reckless, ever ready but never rash. While other men measure out the liquid, fumble about and make a fuss, Simpson, in what an Irishman would call "the most promiscuous manner possible", does the job.

By now Edinburgh was a Mecca for pregnant women, and the docks at the port of Leith were kept busy unloading cargoes

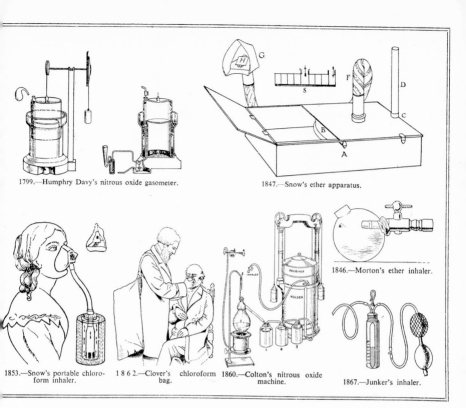

1799.—Humphry Davy's nitrous oxide gasometer.

1847.—Snow's ether apparatus.

1846.—Morton's ether inhaler.

1853.—Snow's portable chloroform inhaler.

1 8 6 2.—Clover's chloroform
bag.

1860.—Colton's nitrous oxide
machine.

1867.—Junker's inhaler.

Early apparatus for
ether and chloroform

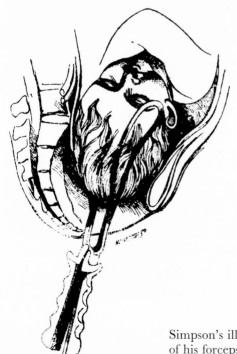

Simpson's illustration showing application
of his forceps

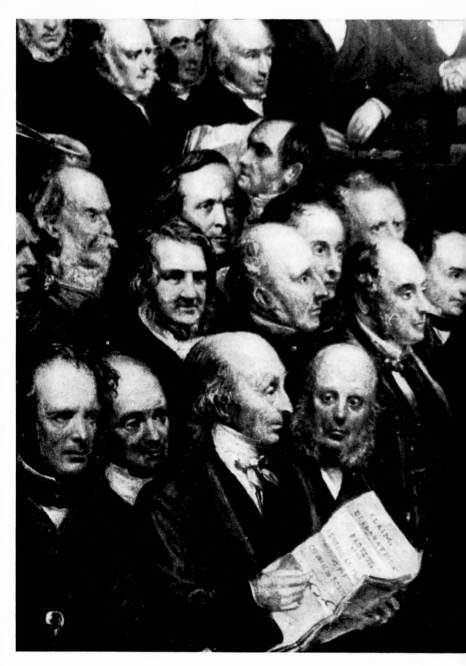

Portion of the painting by D. O. Hill of the 375 men who signed the
Deed of Separation from the Protestant church in 1843. The picture
took so long to complete that many of the subjects are portrayed as
old men!

of ladies from Rotterdam, Le Havre and Copenhagen. Simpson's attraction was his direct approach and his sincerity, and the awakening women of the mid century now, like the Queen, had minds of their own and approved of a doctor who appreciated this and spoke to the point. As has often been quoted, "It is important to be born at the correct time". The women of the mid-nineteenth century were looking for a doctor who would consider them seriously as people, and not baggage. Here was a man who respected women of all classes and considered it their due to receive the best medical attention that there was to offer.

As soon as patients saw Simpson they fell under his charm. But any that he failed to attend were irate. He never forgot a really urgent case; but imaginary ailments he left unattended when overwhelmed by other work. He was deluged with angry letters from these neglected ones; but once he and his patients met, his manner usually disarmed them. "I'll see you in Princes Street", he said to a hypochrondriac who asked when they would meet again "Take a walk there daily in the sun; that is all I can prescribe." Then there was a Lady Helen Ann McKenzie of Rosshaugh in the County Ross, who complained in a correspondence lasting from 1846—1852 that Simpson never arrived for her appointments and failed to answer her letters. In May 1848 she was asking if she should try mustard baths or leeches to relieve the pains in her back, and adds in a P.S. that she is still waiting for the answer to her letter of fully two and a half months ago. In December Simpson wrote a cryptic reply, "Three baths, three leeches", and sent it to the wrong address which further irritated the lady. Seventeen letters passed, until in 1851 her son Henry became ill with headaches and "queer sensations", and Simpson was again badgered for his attention. Also Lady McKenzie was still taking the baths three times a week with no effect. Should she continue? She adds more comment on Simpson's unpardonable behaviour and his lack of response. She moved her boy south to the milder air of Bridge of Allan and eventually Simpson gave in to her repeated entreaties to visit them, and caught the 3.00 a.m. fish train from Edinburgh that ran to Aberdeen.

Simpson was always excited by the railway. He loved the breakneck speed, the sparks striking as the carriages flew along, the clouds of smoke and the demon like noise. On this occasion

F

he travelled in the guard's van along with a London friend,
Dr Marshall Hall who was particularly interested in the nervous
system and is credited with the discovery of the reflex action,
which gave a new insight into the physiology of nerves. The two
men left the train at Stirling and stood in the street to watch the
town welcome a regiment of soldiers from Afghanistan after a
foray in the Kyber Pass, before riding across the valley to
Bridge of Allan. They prescribed white of egg and lime juices for
Henry and left hurriedly in the local doctor's carriage to inpsect
a grave containing Roman coins and a strange medallion, and
returned to Edinburgh by a coach that stopped to allow them
to walk over the field of the battle of Bannockburn where Robert
the Bruce defeated the English host in 1314. Simpson infuriated
his companion by spending $2\frac{1}{2}$ hours grovelling in the turf
searching for arrow tips.

Lady McKenzie was far from satisfied with the visit and wrote
to Simpson bemoaning his short stay. Sh added that "Sir
Banjamin, when attending her husband had stayed $2\frac{1}{2}$ days
and given four long consultations!" A few months later Henry
passed a large worm and recovered, the full credit for which
Lady McKenzie gave Simpson. The letters continued, but
complaint had now been replaced by eulogy.

In the same year Simpson attended the Duchess of Argyll at
Inverary Castle. He was supposed to be there for the birth of
the baby, but arrived too late. The Duke himself had administered chloroform to his wife and was very proud of his success.
Simpson loved Inverary on the shores of misty Loch Fyne.
He would take the train to Glasgow, then the Duke's carriage
along Loch Lomond and over the little pass to the sea at Loch
Long. The road then wound up the long steep Rest and Be
Thankful with Ben-an-Lochan on one side and the Cobbler on
the other. Simpson enjoyed giving a lift to a shepherd and often
remarked that he wished he had the Gaelic and quoted his
friend Christison who had learnt German in two weeks. A
hump backed bridge over the burn was the sign that the
imposing castle was nearly in view and Simpson would put
away his book.

He later reported to his children that Inveraray was a "fairy
tale castle". It still stands on a bank, with wild heights of Ben
Bhuidh behind, and is the most unexpected sight in its surround-

ings. The first glimpse is of the pretty gothic windows of the central tower above the roof-line. Its strange colour gives it a mysterious air of unreality: Simpson described it as being built of blue-green granite with the cones of the slated angle towers stained a deeper green by the weather; the same colour as the bottle glass sheen on the river curling through the trees. The castle is square with a massive battlement tower rising from its heart and dominating the house. It was built in 1746 for the third duke, by Roger Morris and William Adam. Simpson loved the great domed hall, which English travellers have termed "eccentric", and enjoyed the fussiness of the Duchess's boudoir. She had green William Morris wallpaper dotted with lemons and pears and blue forget-me-nots, and an aspidistra in a Minton green fern pot. Simpson admired her French bureau with its green leather inset, and liked to sit on her open-work chair of Indian calamander. Two tall gilt and red Chinese chrysanthemum vases which sat in the window were moved to Simpson's bedroom because he liked them so much.

Up at 6.30 Simpson would walk with the Duke to the watch tower on the top of Duniquoich, immediately above the castle grounds, and look down at the herring fleet on the Loch and the village of Inveraray. This had been planned and laid out for the third Duke by the Scottish architect and engineer, Robert Mylne, when he was working on the interior of the castle, and the austere three-storey terrace houses are quite different from the traditional one-storey cottage of rural Scotland. Simpson remarked that Smollett wrote of the wretched cabins that the Duke's tenants lived in and which clustered round the old castle in the days before 1746. The village church had an entrance at both north and south, and was divided inside into two sections, one for services in English for the Duke of Argyll, and the other in Gaelic for the local people.

Simpson and the Duke would return to the castle after their walk, through the birch scrub by the river, and sit down to a vast breakfast of kidneys, ham and newly-baked baps, served in the Georgian dining room. Robert Mylne considered this interior his finest achievement.

The Argylls enjoyed Simpson's company and always urged him to stay. He particularly admired the Duchess, one reason being that she would not tolerate a wet nurse but always fed her baby herself. "Oh, I love to see a wee bairn cudlin' doon besides its mither," he said, "that's as it should be." He confessed once that he often said that it was difficult to procure a wet nurse, as he could not bear to deny a new baby its own mother's breast.

Usually, though, Simpson was in Edinburgh. Always in a hurry, he never appeared flurried. By 6.00 a.m. he was awake and reading by the gas light in his vast, heavily-carved bed, under a home-made patchwork quilt. At 7.30 the papers arrived—the *Scotsman*, the *Courant* and the *Daily Review*. Having read them, Simpson came downstairs, throwing the newspapers over the banisters in order to have two hands free to carry the pile of books that he had collected for the previous night's reading. He then wrote at the tall, many-drawered desk in his study overlooking the street. Family prayers were at 8.15 in the dining room. Every one had their own Bible in their hand, and the family sat round the mahogany table. Then the six domestic staff were led in by the fat cook, and the rear brought up by the butler. They sat on a form in front of the sideboard, apart from the family. Simpson always read the Lesson, but enjoyed the children leading the prayers. Once this was finished, a great bustle filled the house. Breakfast was at 8.30 and Simpson enjoyed the company of friends as he ate his eggs and bacon, so at least six or eight guests were always present. They were a varied group—archaeologists, foreign doctors, politicians. The Austrian despot, General Haynan, had breakfast at Queen Street during 1849 and so did Winterhalter, the Queen's painter. Just as often, patients sat down to a meal. They would begin to collect at the house by 6.30 a.m. and by 8.30 sixty or more would be waiting. Simpson would exasperate his wife by issuing a loud invitation for "tea and a dish of meal". Some had several hours' carriage journey behind them, and mothers had walked many miles in from the country. After the meal Simpson saw patients in his study. They sat about the house waiting for their turn, overflowing the waiting room, family drawing room and dining room, sitting on the stairs and in the hall. The butler was in charge and no one could talk him into allowing them to jump the queue. Once reproved by an importunate patient who was kept waiting, protesting that he had come to see the doctor all the way from Jedburgh. "Och", replied the butler, "the last one came frae Japan." Simpson would stand at his study door when he was ready for the next patient. He would clap his hands rather than use a bell. "Come away now," would ring down the passage, and the butler would hustle along the next. If several people had arrived at once, they drew lots for priority, the butler standing over them to see fair play.

Simpson's lectures at the University were from 11.00–12.00. and for these he was never late. He returned to Queen Street for lunch at 2.00 always with five or six guests invited on the spur of the moment—artists, lawyers, writers, patients, ministers and doctors, whom he had picked up en route on his journey across town. The rest of the day was crammed with seeing more patients in his own house, treating them in theirs, leaping into his carriage for a dash up the Mound to visit the sick in their tenements of the Old Town, then tearing down the High Street past St Giles and along to the noisy wards of the Lying-in Hospital, Milton House in the Canongate. There were always several people at his heels, and more in his carriage. He invariably carried a book in his hand, his finger keeping the page marked ready for a few moments reading; yet what his patients remembered about him was the undivided attention he gave them. They knew that he was genuinely concerned. Doctors, the few nurses and the patients' relatives rushed to please and the students actually fought to be in the front line to watch his procedures in the hospital ward.

Simpson liked to head for home about 6.00 for a family high tea of bread and ham, fish and custard pudding. Before the table was cleared he would start to romp with the children, rolling on the floor, throwing them into the air, hugging them, smothering them with kisses, hiding in the cupboard in the stair to pounce out with a shriek, turning out the gas lights to play at ghosts or dressing up in the cook's apron and butler's hat. He loved to set a "bogle trap" and roared with laughter when the victim fell in. When the Grindlay relations were present the games were supposed to take on a more sophisticated turn, but Simpson was all for fun. Once when the rest of the party were acting prim scenes of "Rebecca at the Well" and "Flora McDonald waiting for Prince Charlie" he appeared with a learned friend as "The Babes in the Wood" sucking oranges and dressed in frilled pants and pinafores, then lay down on the floor to die, accompanied by roars of laughter from the juveniles in the room. Taking sniffs from the chloroform bottle was another way of turning a genteel party into hilarious fun and the theologian Robert Chalmers' three daughters remember Simpson in the midst of a collection of giggling girls, swooning at his feet in an intoxicated state.

There were now, in 1848, four children, and as many dogs. The youngest child was auburn haired Jessie, fondly called "Sunbeam" by her father. Jessie used to creep through to her father's bed in the night, gazing at him with imploring brown eyes if he tried to move her back to her own. She was not strong and Simpson indulged her, terrified that the gentle merry child would die as Maggie had and break his heart. He poured affection on all his children, but his warm nature was not matched by his wife. Jessie Grindlay disliked the dogs, and spent more and more time by herself in her own room off the living room, reading holy tracts. *The Soul Gatherers* by M. F. Barbour was a favourite. One of her sisters was usually present at 52 Queen Street trying to keep the ineffectual Jessie's head above water. Jessie had begun to find that a little indulgence with the chloroform bottle kept the difficulties of the day away. Simpson was ever tolerant, and his letters to his wife carry no criticism. If he sent her to her parents in Liverpool he organised her journey with the greatest care. He liked people in spite of their shortcomings and never attempted them to change their ways.

In 1848 the family's favourite dog was a Dalmatian called Glen. He would wait for Simpson behind the heavy front door, lurking beside the blue Chinese china umbrella stand, and leap out and bound into the carriage before his master was up the step. He would sit with his head over the side, the wind in his face, as Simpson's carriage always travelled at speed. He expected to go into the patient's house and would stand on the chair beside the bed. Any encouragement from the patient and he would leap in beside her and lick her face. One of the many nursery dogs was Nelson, He was an enormous Newfoundland, with wavy black hair, smooth broad head, silky ears and benevolent face. He put up with the children's mauling though sometimes uttering a blood curdling howl if pulled in two directions at once. He lived on porridge and discarded crusts. "He was very honest," remembers a Simpson child. "When we sat down to eat a piece with Nelson he never took more than his scrimpy allotted share. We took a bite and offered an inch to the anxious-faced dog beside us, who cautiously bit it off by the thumb mark and took the greatest care not to bite the greedy, dirty thumb of the sharer." He was inclined to be over protective, expecially on an outing to the beach at Portobello which was a half-hour drive from town. The big dog assumed territorial rights, would repeatedly swim out to the children with their heavy black leather boots and drop them at their side, to sink to the bottom of the sea. He once went for a plumber who kissed the maid, his snarling white teeth in the big black muzzle having instant effect.

The names and ages of the Simpson dogs were inscribed in a red bound Shakespeare that stood beside the ponderous family bible. Puck, a black and tan terrier, lived at No. 52 for fourteen years. Simpson loved him, although the dog could be wicked, One winter evening, near the end of his days, an extra waiter had been called in to assist Simpson's own man, Jarvis. A dinner party was being held for some visitors from France. This superior, hired waiter soon objected to the little dog constantly under his feet and flipped it with a napkin. Puck took up a dignified stance behind the large brass fender in the dining room, but the waiter bounded him out with a kick. Puck tried to defend himself but was thrown out into the rain and huddled on the well-scrubbed doorstep till the guests arrived. At last they all sat down round the mahogany table, but the new waiter was a disaster. He spilled the soup and his usually steady hands jerked as he served the entrée. The gravy dish slid on its saucer and the waiter walked with the trailing step of an American slave. Spasms passed over his normally immobile face and every time he stood close to the table he was noticed to shudder and twitch. Simpson and his children realized what was up and tried to oust the little dog with the snapping teeth from under the folds of the voluminous cream lace table-cloth, but he carried on his guerrilla warfare successfully until the ladies moved upstairs and coffee was brought in. Puck had a rather ugly daughter called Kelp who also lived at "52" Simpson sat fondling her elephant-like ears one evening, and contrasted them to Puck's smart head. The idea crossed his mind that cropping Kelp's "lugs" would make her more like her handsome father. Five of Simpson's colleagues were present, and they urged him on, all promising help. The terrier followed her easy-going master trustingly into the study. Simpson insisted on chloroform and the dog was soon under the spell. The six doctors tried their hand at docking the velvet ears, but after much snipping and cutting they had to give up in order to save the mutilated dog from an anaesthetic death! Simpson preserved the bits of ears in a bottle of spirit which he kept on the mantelpiece. If a sarcastic guest enquired, "And where are your dog's ears?" Simpson would suppress the banter by answering, "Did you wish to see them?" and produce the horrible remains.

The Simpson children were very evident in the house. No banishing to a nursery flat for them. They played Arabs in the big hall, using umbrellas for tents, and the two flights of stairs made hide-and-seek a great game. The children were only rebuked if they disturbed a country patient still resting in a back room. Anxious relatives would lurk on the back stairs waiting to trap Simpson if he ran down, as he often did, for a quick cup of tea and slice of thick brown bread. Jarvis insisted on serving this from a massive silver tray, a present for services rendered in producing an heir to Blenheim Castle.

There was something childlike in Simpson's character, which perhaps explains his popularity with children. One little girl, who later married into the family, remembers standing at the big Georgian window of her home in the old town on the West side of George Square, waiting for Simpson to visit her mother. She gazed out at the newly planted rhododendrons in the Square gardens, and at last heard the swift-steeping horses clattering furiously over the cobbles and the wheels of the carriage skidding round the right corner. She dashed downstairs to open the door and see the dogs springing out of the brougham. The doctor seldom had to ring. He climbed the stairs, slowly loosening his sealskin coat, passing a stuffed eagle and on through the red door to her mother's room asking kindly all the way as to her progress. Simpson had time to enjoy the joke when a huge doll was carried in first when the new baby was rung for, and with his big arm round the child would draw her to his knee, fishing in his pocket for a trinket, saying to the nurse "plenty of fresh butter is as good as cod liver oil".

Another child, L. B. Walford, later wrote of him in her *Recollections of a Scottish Novelist*.

Simpson attended my mother in all her serious illnesses; and one day, on leaving her room at Portobello. his nostrils were assailed by a powerful and delicious odour. He snuffed it up, and pronounced without hesitation, "I smell toffee. Toffee's very wholesome . . ." The enchanted toffee-makers surrounded their enlightened friend and protector like a swarm of bees; he had more of it pressed upon him than he knew what do do with; his dictum was our joy and bulwark forever after.

Dear little fat "Simmy"; we owed him much . . . apart from toffee. He was neither too grand nor too busy to attend us in our childish ailments, confident that he would not have been sent for if another would have done; and when I was eleven years old one of these summonses was sent on my behalf. I had an abscess in both ears from bathing in the sea too late in the season, and had been hurried into Edinburgh from Oban by my anxious parents . . . Part of the journey was made by steamboat and I lay in my berth as still as a stone; a few hours later, when I awoke to consciousness, there was a sense of something warm, soft, heavy and suffocatingly close, hanging over me. It was "Simmy" putting on leeches! It was in the middle of the night, but he had come on the instant; and as the little patient was sleeping, he applied his leeches without waking her; finally forgetting his proportions in the ardour of his task, he well-nigh smothered her. But he brought her through.

Simpson always carried a narrow-brimmed hat, which he wore well back, showing his whole face and part of his head. His suit was black, but he wore a nicely arranged white neckpiece, with a very carefully made bow in the front, and he rather enjoyed a coloured waistcoat. He dressed with the same care for a night call, and it was seldom that he had an uninterrupted sleep. A speaking trumpet led from the front door to a servant's bed in the basement but it was usually Simpson himself who answered the bell, up and ready in a flash.

At Queen Street he could never escape the ring at the door and the constant demand from the patients. His solution was to buy a little house in Trinity, then a village a few miles away from the town, overlooking the Firth of Forth. Called View-bank, it was a small square house with roses all round. Simpson loved the place and would drive down in the sunset from the grey town to tend the garden for a few hours. He planted lilac, laburnum and apple trees in groups on the grass, and masses more roses, particularly white. His neighbours were the fishermen of Newhaven, and Simpson enjoyed their unsophisticated company, so like that of the independent weavers of his childhood days. He liked to repay their friendship by attending their wives, and his direct "Come away, now what's this that's wrong?" was a sound a sick woman liked to hear. They were strong people, up before dawn gutting the fish, then walking into town with creels on their backs. Their bare feet slapped on the cobbles as their shouts rang out on the empty early morning streets—"Wha'll buy my herrin'?" Their blue and white stripped skirts over many petticoats and their trim waisted blouses would be seen at the foot of the tenement stairs or at the door of the terraced houses in the squares. Simpson often attended the Newhaven Free Church, crammed with the fishermen, and he joined in the unaccompanied psalms with a lusty drone. He was friendly with the minister, Mr Fairbairn, who was struggling to establish more food shops in the village, and less drink.

Tea, an egg and an undisturbed sleep was all that Simpson asked of Viewbank, and he was known to creep down silently and hide his tell-tale hat so that no one knew that he was there. 'My een are gone t' gither with sleep", he said to his coachman more than once as he stumbled through the gate. It was a good starting place, too, for his antiquarian excursions to the islands in the Firth; Inchcolm with its hermit cell he visited time and time again, and the marked stones at Inchkeith.

Simpson was satisfied with his environment and genuinely happy with the challenge of his work. He felt no need to uproot himself when in the spring of 1848 he received several letters from a leading London obstetrician, Prothero Smith, enticing him with offers of the midwifery wards at St Bartholomew's Hospital, London. Smellie, Hunter, Liston and many others had been lured south and, on Liston's sudden death, Syme himself had accepted his position at the University College Hospital. Boswell quoted Johnston as saying "the best and busiest road in Scotland is the one leading south" and Simpson was further tempted by a letter from the entire staff of St Bartholomew's inviting him "as one whose abilities and skill have gained for him the highest professional character" to accept the Midwifery Chair.

Prothero Smith hoped for the position himself, but declared that he would not apply if there was any chance of Simpson accepting. Smith was out of favour with the London Establishment at the moment, as he had written to the Lancet and lay Press asking why no fitting "testimonial" had yet been given by the medical profession to the discoverer of the anaesthetic properties of chloroform, and chiding the doctors, en masse, for this lapse.

However, Simpson had no difficulty in declining the offer, answering the letter on the day that he received it. European and American doctors, and even the Queen, came north, he wrote, therefore why "should he consider abandoning Scotland when London had nothing to offer him that he did not have himself?" People were more important to him than wealth, and he was far too sentimental to cast aside his country and his friends.

Scotland had, in fact, become respectable. The Queen had taken a lease of Balmoral House the previous year, and her subjects knew from her the joys of spending the day in the rain on a pony, and night in an earth floored stone bothy like Alt na Guithasach, then striding out towards the top of the hill in the clear air, with the view to the glen unfolding below. Prince Albert would build a cairn on the summit and jump on the top to give three loud cheers, while the ghillie came up with the picnic hamper on the pony's back. The Queen actually preferred Scotland to England, and everything Scottish had suddenly become fashionable. Paperweights of Balmoral granite were much in demand, and tartan, reels, bagpipes and sporrans were considered cultured and refined where before they had been hidden away with the whisky bottle when friends from the South arrived.

At the time of Prothero Smith's offer Simpson was deep

in a new project, and on 28 December 1848 he stunned the Edinburgh Obstetrical Society with a paper crititled "Vacuum Extraction—a Substitute for Forceps in Tedious Labour".

The forceps of the Chamberlen family had gone far in helping to extract the baby when the mother could not push it out herself, but often the baby's head was squashed or the mother herself injured by the brutal metal blades. Twelve years before, in the summer of 1836, Simpson had hit on an ingenious alternative. Suck the baby out! The idea had crossed his mind when, walking along an Edinburgh street with a friend, Robert Paterson. They had passed a group of boys playing "suckers". They were seeing who could lift the largest stone with a piece of wet leather threaded with a string. He watched for a while, then joined in the game.

The principle was not original. As Simpson quoted in his paper, James Young, a naval surgeon and mayor of Plymouth, recorded details in 1694 of a prolonged labour where "a cupping glass fixed to the scalp with an air pump failed to bring out the head". In 1706 it failed him again, and Young dropped the idea. Previously Pare had used a cupping glass to raise depressed fractures of the skull, and in 1665 suggested the glass could be useful in war wounds to draw splinters to the surface. In 1794 Saemann of Jena wrote, "I saw in a dream an air pump wherewith one can seize the head of an infant without injury to the mother or child. The pump was made of brass and had a covering of rubber with ventilators". However, he never put his dream into effect! An Aberdeen graduate, Neil Arnott, who practised in London and helped found London University along with Lord Brougham and the Queen's physician James Clark, published in 1829 a study called *Elements of Physics* in which he stated that "a pneumatic tractor *might* be useful as a substitute for the steel forceps, in the hands of a man deficient in manual dexterity".

Arnott never carried his theory farther than a diagram, but Simpson followed up his idea. How do limpets stick to rocks? he asked himself How do lamprey eels hang on? What makes a cuttlefish attach itself to its prey? How does a leech work? Having considered these questions over several years, Simpson wrote to a friend,

I have been up for three nights working . . . I will enclose in this two tractors, the instrument is now nearly perfect. I showed it last Wednesday to the Medico Chirurgical Society. There was a great crowd etc. The experiments went off beautifully. I fixed a small tractor in the palm of my right hand before them, and lifted up with it an iron weight of 28 lbs. It could lift double. One of the physicians of the St Petersburg Court is here. He admired the "idea" but doubted if it would really answer in practice. Well, I took him and others down a few days ago to the Hospital to see a badish case, and fixed the tractor on. The operation was most successful. The Russian danced with joy, crying *"C'est superbe, superbe; c'est immortalitié à vous"*.

Simpson's instrument consisted of a round metal spectrum fitted over a piston, with a large handle to enable a good practical grip. The broader trumpet-shaped end was covered with leather and greased with lard, and this was then applied to the foetal head. It could also be applied to the baby's bottom, and could then draw the child down until it was in a position to be turned safely.

Reservations came quickly from colleagues and the medical press. One of the first letters in the *Lancet* read, "We almost dread the infant's scalp being torn off and the parietal bone dragged out." The usual controversy flared up, and with it came numerous voices claiming exclusive invention of the apparatus. A Dr James, Mayor of Exeter in 1828, reported that he had independently drawn an instrument to suck out the placenta and James Mitchell, a student in Simpson's '47 class wrote that he had made a diagram of an instrument after watching Simpson's fail, and that he had written this up in his examination paper. Simpson answered calmly that he had never actually seen those papers—his assistant had marked them— and that anyway his ultimate design was based on the "artificial leech of Guidicelli, consisting of a suction apparatus around a dark that he used to pierce the skin".

In January 1849 Simpson wrote, "I have now employed [the tractor] repeatedly when the head was above the brim, and already sunk into the pelvic cavity". His assistants were using the instrument, and his students writing up the results. Doctors in Paris, Dublin and London asked for the design and then sent back enthusiast reports. Simpson's old correspondent, Dr Sharpey, added in his letter on the subject "What is to become of our redundant population? The sanitary people on one hand keeping folks from dying and you with your chloroform and other 'contraps' smoothing the road into the world; it will be like the threatened glut of gold and reduce the value of honest people . . . Henceforth you must be told to take care of yourself, because good folk are scarce!"

Simpson was aware of the defects of the instrument, and tried modifications and improvements. He experimented with cow hide instead of pig skin, and even horse, to make the cup less flexible and so prevent it slipping on the child's head and releasing the vacuum. By 1850 he had abandoned the idea, and had turned again to the conventional forceps which he tried to adapt to his needs. However, in a paper published in the *London Medical Gazette*, he predicted that "the construction of the air tractor is still very far from being so perfect as it will yet be rendered", and he foresaw it displacing the forceps from the obstetrician's armamentarium completely. Little did he know that by 1954 a Swedish designed "Vacuum extractor", based exactly on his principles but using materials unavailable in 1849, would be gaining acceptance in the labour wards in Scandinavia. Today this "Malström" instrument is used on the Continent, in England and the U.S.A. and in the more modern maternity units in Simpson's own Scotland as a first choice by the obstetrician. The instrument is now more sophisticated, with a flexible tube to enable it to be drawn around a corner, and with the ability to control the pressure exerted on the baby's head. It is far less painful to the mother than forceps and much gentler to the baby and makes the interminable wait for the anaesthetist unnecessary; as Simpson would have said, "it is a kinder instrument altogether". A modern obstetrical professor and authority on the subject states: "I acknowledge priority to Simpson in the effective application of a vacuum to the presenting part of a foetus for the purpose of affixing a traction device to aid delivery . . . There are far less reports of inter-cranial complications when it is used . . . as it is impossible to succeed if one is rough in one's technique, it is a great factor for mother and child." The modern doctor is inclined to look at Simpson's instrument and say that it is impossible to use, but it must be remembered that the same is said today of the earliest skis, the original microscope; and how many of us can cope with a "penny farthing"? In Simpson's hands his device did work as his contemporaries reported and grateful Victorian mothers carefully recorded in their diaries.

Simultaneously with developing the extractor, Simpson was modifying the design of the traditional forceps. He set up his own forge in the basement at Queen Street, and his wife complained in a letter to her sister that the cook had left because of "the noise, the sparks and the smell". Simpson first demonstrated his modification to the Edinburgh Obstetrical Society in May 1848. In his design, as he explained, the blades were longer than before and differed in that

"the shanks are parallel for some distance beyond the lock, an indispensable point in order to prevent them injuring the outlet; in their blades being curved: and in the part intended to embrace the head being sufficiently long and large. . . . The blades are the same as Dr F. Ramsbotham's, but scarcely so much curved. The lock is Smellie's but with knees or projections above it of such size as to prevent the blades readily unlocking in the intervals between the pains, these giving it the fixed character of the locks of Levret and Bunninghausen's instruments, without their complexity. The joints are made so loose as to allow of their lateral motion and overlapping to a very considerable degree, thus facilitating their introduction and application. And, lastly, the handle is that used by Naegele and other German accoucheurs, viz. with transverse knees or rests below the lock for one or two of the first fingers of the right hand to drag by, the long forceps being only properly used as an instrument of traction, not of compression. In addition, the handles are grooved and marked on the anterior side, to distinguish that from the other side when the blades are within the pelvis. . . .

Simpson felt that the use of his forceps was indicated by a deformed pelvis on the mother's part, resulting in the child's head having to be turned before it could be born. He wrote in the September *Journal of Medical Science*, 1848:

The blades of the long forceps should be placed obliquely upon the child's head,—one, the posterior, over the side of the occiput; and the other, or anterior, over the side of the brow or temple, and consequently, should be situated in the oblique diameter of the brim—the markings on the child's head after birth always show this mode of application of the instrument; when properly applied upon the mother, and when their situation relative to the pelvis is examined, they are found to have assumed this position; and in experiments with the instrument (when the head of a dead child is fixed in a pelvis with a contracted brim), this is the position and relation which the instrument will be seen to assume with relation to the infantile head and maternal pelvis. Besides, in thus placing the instrument, while we incur less danger of injuring the urethra and other important parts, we place the blades of the instrument in exactly those parts of the pelvic circle where there is least pressure and consequently most room for them. . . .

These forceps soon became the standard instrument for dealing with difficult "cephalic presentations". Simpson's nephew, Alexander, later modified the design as did various obstetricians in the early 1900s but nowadays these modifications have been discarded, and the basic instrument used in most maternity hospitals is Simpson's own. A current American obstetrical textbook illustrates Simpson's forceps as the standard model. They are uncomplicated and easy to use having a handle that can be readily grasped, with notches for the fingers to prevent a slip.

No wonder Simpson wrote to his sister Mary at this time, "I hunger for a book, and I thirst for time to read it". In the following year, 1850, Simpson was elected President of the Edinburgh Royal College of Physicians. Charles II had issued the Patent to erect the Royal College in 1681 and since then the Fellows had provided medical care for the poor. In 1704 the College acquired a hall in Fountain Close and there two physicians ran a dispensary on three afternoons a week. The College looked upon this as a serious obligation, and any Fellow who did not attend at the specified hours was fined, the money being used to buy medicines for the patients. Treatment was hampered by the lack of any hospital beds, which led to an appeal in 1725 which, together with the help of the new Lord Provost, George Drummond, successfully launched the Edinburgh Royal Infirmary. The Royal College was closely involved with the University, and laid down the rules to maintain the standard that a student must reach before practising medicine. The office of President of the College carried much authority and Simpson was very flattered to be chosen "an honour which I confess I greatly value, not only because it is the highest honour to which a Scottish physician can possibly aspire, but also because I was elected to it (and I believe elected unanimously) by the free votes of my fellow practitioners; and that too at an age when the office has been conferred upon few". He would be happy to know that his own library now rests under the College roof in Queen Street, not far along the street from his own house at No. 52.

The Royal College was a meeting place for the leading physicians of the town. There was much for them to talk about at the approach of the mid-century. The loudest conversations circled round the fact that the Irish were starving. Instead of arousing sympathy in Edinburgh, this caused alarm, and the papers were full of foreboding. It was considered that boatloads of riff-raff wouldl be sailing up the Clyde, and, finding no work in the already over-populated Glasgow, the rabble would wend it way east and end up causing trouble in the seething lands of the Old Town. The worthy citizens of Edinburgh were worried that, rather than potatoes, the Irish mob would find ale, and the substitute was always disastrous!

There was no mention in the Edinburgh press that the atrocious famine conditions in Ireland were due to the land policy of the British Government, which, when the potato crops failed, did nothing effective to alleviate the misery of the people. During the two centuries before the famine the Irish had been dispossessed of their lands by the landed gentry of England who had been given it for services rendered to the Crown. Through the years, the people on the land became broken in spirit, feckless and irresponsible, and now, leaving Ireland in their hordes and arriving destitute in Glasgow, with nothing to live on, they took to drink as a means of temporary oblivion from the unalloyed misery of their lot.

Turning to a more cheerful subject, the physicians would talk about that peculiar girl, Elizabeth Blackwell, who had just arrived in Liverpool from America, clutching, of all things, a medical degree! Championing the bizarre, *Punch* carried seven stanzas in her honour, a couple of which ran:

> Young ladies all of every clime,
> Especially of Britain,
> Who wholly occupy your time
> In novels or in knitting
> Whose highest skill is but to play
> Sing, dance, or French to clack well,
> Reflect on the example, pray,
> of Excellent Miss Blackwell!

> For Doctrix Blackwell—that's the way
> To dub in rightful gender
> In her profession, ever may
> Prosperity attend her!
> Punch, a gold handled parasol
> Suggests for presentation
> To one so well deserving all
> Esteem and admiration.

Expecting a grim and masculine woman, the country, and particularly the doctors, were dumbfounded to discover that Elizabeth was young and pretty. Most members of the Royal College of Physicians treated Miss Blackwell as a good joke, but Simpson did not laugh at her, or *Punch;* on thinking it over, he decided that women could become very useful doctors, and should be helped to do so, and publicly stated that he would like to meet Miss Blackwell, and wish her luck.

Another woman was under discussion, but this one was black. Harriet Tubman was an escaped slave from Maryland. Instead of fleeing to Canada and British protection, she had washed dishes in Philadelphia and managed to save some money out of her pitiful wage; then, alone and travelling only at night, she went back to Maryland to lead her sister and two children north to freedom. Over the next ten years she returned again and again to the South, and helped more than 300 slaves escape. Her weapons were an old pistol to fend off pursuers and a rag soaked in opium to stuff into crying babies' mouths. Rewards as high as £12,000 were posted for her capture. Once over the Ohio river, she transported her charges North in covered farm wagons, and in loads of lumber, and once lined twenty-eight of them up as a funeral procession and walked them slowly and southerly to safety. Frederick Douglass was another name linked with the slave question. Simpson began to attend church more regularly in order to hear a particular, Free Church Minister who championed the abolitionist cause and in 1846 Presbyterian admirers had made Douglass legally free by paying his Maryland master £150. They began to regret this when they realised that Douglass was asking not only for freedom but demanding black equality as well, including the right to vote! This was considered outrageous.

Nearer to home, the Edinburgh conversation often turned to Harry Goodsir, the brother of Simpson's colleague, John Goodsir, who had succeeded the maligned Knox in anatomy. Harry had sailed with Sir John Franklin on his last voyage in search of the North-West Passage. H.M.S. *Terror* and *Erebuos* had left the Thames on 18 May 1845. The ships' last contact with civilisation was along the north-west coast of Greenland where they met the whaler, *Prince of Wales*, on 26 July 1845. The *Erebus* and *Terror* exchanged greetings and Captain Dannet, the whaler's master, reported in his log that both crews were well and in remarkable spirits, expecting to finish the operation in good time. Crossing Baffin Bay, the two ships entered Lancaster Sound, slowly sailing into oblivion.

Closely associated with the *Erebus* and *Terror* was another colleague of Simpson, Sir John Richardson; he sailed with the first relief ship that set off in 1848 and spent two years in a fruitless search for Franklin. He came to Edinburgh and stayed at 52 Queen Street when writing up the zoological discoveries made on his voyage, in a great four-volume work.

Then there was that reckless Palmerston to talk about, who was involving the country in European wars; to say nothing of Prince Albert and the glass pavilions that he was setting up in Hyde Park. Simpson visited London at this time and wrote home, "We saw the spot where King Charles was beheaded. I

have been an hour in the British Museum, revelling in some
Roman antiquities. I saw Prince Albert yesterday; very kind
and gentlemanly; showed me his library, etc.; talked of *Punch*,
Scotland and chloroform. I went over the Palace, and was
introduced to the Prince of Wales, Prince Alfred, and the two
youngest children."

Simpson was forced to return hurriedly from London, as he
was feeling ill, and he arrived back in Edinburgh at the same
time as his letter. A poisoned finger had led to an ugly abscess in
his axilla. Blood poisoning was a common cause of death in
these days, but Simpson was reluctant to do anything about his
infection. His assistants persuaded Jessie, however, that a
surgeon *must* be called in. James Miller was deeply hurt that he
had not been asked. Simpson did assure him, but not till four
years later, that he himself would have consulted Miller, but
that his wife moved faster than him on this occasion. She
summoned Syme!

As we have seen, Syme and Simpson had been antagonists
from the beginning. They had argued on the same side over the
quashing of the homoepathists, but otherwise they made a
point of opposing each other on every issue that arose.

Syme had moved to London on Liston's sudden death in
1847, the result of the boom from his yacht hitting his chest.
Syme was appointed to Liston's chair in London, but five
months later he was back in Edinburgh. The students at the
London University Hospital had objected to Syme's succession
and had demonstrated publicly against the professors responsible for his appointment. Syme said he could not work in this
atmosphere, under such conditions. He also complained that
the London doctors were so busy running after their private
patients and their money, that no one had time to talk or think!
Also he "Feared for his children's sake, the want in London of
the free air and exercise they always enjoyed in Charlotte
Square and at his suburban villa at Millbank" (below the
Blackford Hill). Millbank was indeed lovely, with fruit trees and
glass houses among which Syme's daughter Alice was later
courted by a bright young assistant of Syme's, a Joseph Lister,
who took her away to Glasgow as his bride.

Syme was now considered one of the foremost surgeons in
Europe. He had been born at 56 Princes Street, the son of a

rather peculiar, obstinate Edinburgh lawyer. He attended the
Edinburgh Royal High School, and was taught by Professor
Pillans, who later had Simpson in his class when he afterwards
became Professor of Humanity at the University. Syme learnt
from Robert Christison's father, but his main interest was in
chemistry.

At the age of sixteen he had discovered a way of waterproofing cloth by dissolving caoutchouc in coal tar, and his
method was adopted by the Glasgow manufacturer, Mr
MacIntosh. As a schoolboy, Syme had been persuaded by his
friend Liston, already a young surgeon, to study medicine. He
became particularly interested in anatomy, and in 1822 he
visited Paris where bodies were readily available for dissection.
Here he lodged in a cheap hotel with another young graduate,
Dr Sharpey of London and so cemented a life-long association.
Syme returned to become a clerk in the Edinburgh Royal
Infirmary. At that time bleeding was the remedy for everything, but Syme questioned the usefulness of this treatment, and
became very unpopular by refusing to draw twelve ounces of
blood from the arm of a dying boy. He ordered "porter and beef
steak" instead, but was overruled; his superior believing that a
"generous diet would only feed the disease and make it worse".
The blood was drawn and the boy died.

Now, however, Syme was in an unassailable position, and
treated his patients as he thought fit. Called in by Jessie, he
dealt efficiently with his unexpected patient, and for the time
being the two men were friends. Syme even admitted to Simpson that he now took back all that he had said against anaesthetics. It is interesting to note, however, that even as late as
1861 Syme expected his patients to endure severe pain, surely
unnecessarily. A student in Syme's clinical surgery class,
William McNeil, wrote in his notebook:

21st Nov. 1861. Case 12 was that of an old surly-looking
fellow, who was brought in, suffering from a very rare disease
north of the Tweed, viz. Chimney Sweeper's Cancer on
Scrotum. When asked by Pr. Syme if he had ever been South
of the Tweed, he said in a very surly tone, "Aye, I hae been
in Perth". "Had he ever swept chimneys?" "Na!" When
asked if he would take chloroform or not, he made no reply.

Pr. Syme with a pair of scissors at once cut out the cancer which was situated on the most dependent part of the scrotum. The shouts of the old fellow were terrific. Pr. Syme, after he had completed the tying of the vessel cut, questioned him concerning the period of its growth, and got for a reply: "Hoo the devil can I answer ony questions just noo?" This created a very hearty laugh among the students, which did not improve the temper of the patient. He left the theatre uttering imprecations on Pr. Syme and all concerned.

Syme told Simpson that when he first entered the theatre to watch Miller operating on a patient under ether, there were so many Free Church ministers present that Syme "doubted whether he had not intruded upon a meeting of the Presbytery!" Syme was Professor of Clinical Surgery in Edinburgh for thirty-six years and some of his operations are classics in the art of surgery. An amputation at the ankle joint is called after him and its success in 1842 enabled many patients to retain at least most of their limb. He gave two clinical lectures a week, operated on three days a week and spent about two hours in the hospital each morning. He operated very precisely, without the flamboyant showmanship of Liston. He hardly spoke to his assistants. They were supposed to know exactly what to do. Dr John Brown wrote of Syme that "he never wasted a word, or a drop of ink, or a drop of blood".

He was no friend of Simpson's neighbour, James Miller, a much gentler man. Well known as an orator, Miller was much involved with the Disruption of the Church in 1843. He was on the side of the Free Church and did much for its cause by speech and publications. He was also a great champion of temperance reform. His lectures on surgery were very popular with the students; full of anecdotes and flashes of wit, and on any excuse, tirades against drink. His book, *System of Surgery*, had a great sale in America, and was responsible for Edinburgh techniques being adopted by such influential people as Dr Warren and Dr Bigelow in Massachusetts. Fourteen years ahead of time, in 1864, Miller felt that he was dying and went to see Syme in his home. Syme was standing in front of the fire with his hands behind his back. Miller, thin and emaciated, held out his hand, saying he had come to say goodbye. "Huh", said Syme, "so you've come to apologise have you? Well, I forgive ye", and turned away.

With Syme's expert treatment Simpson gradually recovered, although he was dangerously ill for some weeks. When convalescing, he was persuaded by Syme to take a holiday. He reluctantly agreed, and went over to Holland by boat from Leith, then, as he described it, "scampered" round the German, Belgian and French universities. Europe had changed since his previous visit. There had been revolutions in Germany and Italy, and France was a republic once more. Simpson wrote from Paris to his sister-in-law.

Paris 23rd April 1850.

Dear Isobel,

I have just written a note to Jessie. What subject shall I scribble on for you?

Let me begin by saying that, to a stranger, like myself, Paris is a far far more remarkable place than London with its numerous and gigantic palaces and fountains, its high high and narrow streets, its beautiful gardens, its gay and light scene and its inhabitants. Some of the buildings are superb. I was at the top of the Parthum before breakfast—a superb view of the city with no smoke covering it as in London or Edinburgh but the sun glistening on its endless white houses and the Seine—I went to the church of St Racquel. The service was fearfully, fearfully Catholic with priests in the gayest possible gowns, long candles burning, men throwing around perfume, bells ringing, women busily busily uttering prayers and men holding out everywhere dishes with holy water for you to touch.

After dining for 20 pence in a choice of 10 or 70 dishes we went out to one of the gates of the City to see how the middle and lower orders spend their Sunday evening. There were 6 or 8 balls going on in a gushet beyond the gate. In one I counted above 100 persons dancing at once and perhaps 300 watching them. Is thus our Edinburgh strange? Shops all shut at 10 or 11? But my letter is done—my arm is wearied.

J. Y. S.

In Bonn, Simpson was invited to watch an operation on a woman suffering from the dreaded complication of a long delivery; a vesico vaginal fistula. The operation was unsuccessful. Simpson then spent an evening arguing with a Professor Martin of Jena, about why patients died after an amputation, and discussing how chloroform lowered the incidence of death (Martin had cut down fatalities among his patients from 70 per cent to 35 per cent). There is no record of Simpson lecturing abroad on this occasion. His aim was to learn, not to teach. He was particularly interested in European surgical instruments, and had many of his own made abroad. A watchmaker in Bonn made forceps and silver sutures for him, but Simpson complained that "although his workmanship was great, he was a poor man at getting the job done, and needed 3 or 4 letters before he sent the article". Simpson paid him by sending half of a £5 note in the first letter, and the other half in the last. The instrument under discussion in 1850 was the stethescope.

It had been discovered by Laennec in 1816, who was called in to see a patient who was so fat that the doctor could not hear her heart. Remembering seeing two children playing with a log of wood, and so sending messages to each other, Laennec rolled up a sheet of paper and held it with one end to his ear, and the other on the patient's chest.

Previously, Hippocrates, who apparently knew everything, had described laying his ear on the patient's chest and hearing "creakings as of leather", but, as Laennec said, "the old way was was not only ineffective, but inconvenient, indelicate and, in hospitals, even disgusting". His so-called stethescope was a cylinder of wood, half an inch in diameter and one foot long, with a hole hollowed out into a funnel shape at one end. Simpson took the Edinburgh version of the new instrument to Bonn with him in 1850, but the doctors there were very scathing, and said they could hear much better with their own. Actually Simpson agreed with them, as he later confessed to his students but, always the patriot he "did not let on".

In Germany Simpson saw the outstanding German pathologist, Robert Virchow, who was also an antiquarian and anthropologist with a particular interest in old lake dwellings. Simpson told him of the vitrified fort built in a little lake on the east side of Loch Fyne, that he had been shown a few years previously by the Duke of Argyll. Virchow had been banished from Berlin for a while because he publicly blamed an epidemic of typhus on deplorable housing conditions, and put forward the revolutionary idea that it was the State's responsibility to do something about it. Simpson was crystallising his own ideas on contagion at this time. Virchow was working on his theory regarding cells as the ultimate unit of diseased tissues, and the German dedicated his book on the subject in 1858, to Simpson's friend, John Goodsir, as a tribute to Goodsir's "acute observations on cell life".

On his "scamper" in Europe Simpson came across a telescope. Returning home, he decided that he wanted one on the roof of Viewbank. He asked for advice from Scotland's authority on the subject, Sir William Keith Murray, and also from the Dublin occulist William Wilde, whose son Oscar is perhaps better remembered.

Simpson and William Wilde found that they had much in common. Wilde was an antiquarian, and the two men were enthusiastic about each other's finds. Wilde was particularly interested in Simpson's work on old leper houses, and unearthed much information about those on Irish soil. He excavated several sites in Sligo and Kerry to discover the cause of death of the mummified remains. Ireland was the land of the cromlech, a large flat stone supported by three upright stones, and Wilde described 780 of them, including one of 120 feet wide. His favourite one was a few miles from Drogheda, near the battle-field of the Boyne, and years later, in 1857, Wilde took Simpson to see it. The large tomb was situated in the midst of one of the greatest cemeteries of Pagan Ireand, with twenty smaller cromlechs on all sides. To reach the tomb, one had to stoop through a narrow doorway into a totally dark passage sixty-two feet long. In some places it was possible to walk upright, at others to squeeze through on hands and knees. The stones forming the walls were five to eight-feet high, standing on their ends, and the roof was made of flagstones of great size. The passage led into a cavern, with a lofty domed roof. Three other chambers led off, forming the shape of a cross, and on the floor of each was a stone basin. Wilde likened this tomb to the Pyramids, which he had visited. Simpson later became very interested in the size of the Pyramids and repeatedly wrote to Wilde and asked for his first-hand impressions.

Wilde now told Simpson that he feared the weather in Scotland was too wet by far for an amateur telescope, but Sir William Keith Murray was more helpful. He sent Simpson "charts, globes, 25 books on astronomy and a sketch of a telescope with notes on its manipulation which may appear trifling but are nevertheless essential in practice". In these notes Murray stresses the need for a steady stand and, more important, a steady hand. Murray later visited Viewbank and drew up a detailed plan of what was needed to set up Simpson's observatory.

Optics intrigued Simpson, as did the new-fangled camera. His assistant was particularly interested in photography, as was his friend Dr Octavius Hill, who is now remembered as a master of the art. Simpson sent his sister Mary, who was just moving from Tasmania to the mainland of Australia, a photograph of himself for Christmas. He wrote in the covering letter that it would be easy to carry "and probably you would value it at times as a remembrance of a rascal who owes his dearest sister so very, very much". This photograph was taken in a little wooden hut at the foot of the Mound. The photographer later remembered Simpson rushing in, saying "Come away, quickly now". He searched for some small money in his coat pocket, but, unable to find any, handed over a £5 note, and told the photographer to send the change along with the likeness to 52 Queen Street. With his coat unbuttoned and his long curly hair flying, he rushed out and off.

In 1850 the Edinburgh Royal Infirmary took the unprecedented step of appointing Simpson as "an extra physician for the diseases of women and infants". Specialisation was beginning to obtain a foothold in the hospital, and a ward only for diseases of the eye was opened at this time. The Infirmary laid down the rule that a patient allocated to Simpson was "not to be placed in that ward until she has been made aware by the Matron that she will be under the charge of the said physician and may be more particularly the subject of attention to the lecturer and the students than she might be in a general ward". Simpson's appointment was not made in connection with the Chair of Midwifery, but as a personal tribute to his work in the subject of diseases of women. This was the first public gesture of appreciation in his home town. Honours were slow to come to Simpson. In 1853 he received a letter from two former students now in London, who wanted to take up a public subscription as an acknowledgement of his "most important discovery of this age", but Simpson asked them not to carry their idea any further. In 1857 he received a letter from France from a friend of Lord Brougham, urging him to "tell the public of the part you have played in the matter of chloroform" as so few people knew.

A letter of a different colour appeared in the *Lancet* of September 1851. The editor, Dr Wakley, explained afterwards that he was on holiday by the sea and it had been "slipped in" without his knowledge. The letter was headed "Obstetric Quackery in Edinburgh" and was signed Isaac Irons, M.D. It was a damning attack on Simpson's methods of treatment. It accused him of "rushing unnecessarily into the operation of Caesarian Section" and of using "infernal and appalling machines" to retain a retroverted uterus. Also it accused Simpson of "encouraging the practise of homoepathy and mesmerism and of being quite unworthy of the position as President of the Royal College of Physicians".

Simpson challenged the letter, publishing a somewhat scathing reply in the *Lancet* for 29 September. He claimed to know Irons' identity because "There is in the medical profession only *one* individual who does use, on professional subjects, language so indiscreet as that of the well-known writer in question; and, that after all, this individual was scarcely legally responsible for his own outbreaks of violence".

Isaac Irons was Dr Robert Lee, born in Melrose, Roxburgh, and a graduate of Edinburgh. He was now a noted London obstetrician who had contributed some original work on the nerves of the uterus, and whose book *Clinical Midwifery* was widely read. According to Simpson, patients had come to him from London as they objected to Lee's "indelicate treatment". This in turn was denied by Irons, who insisted in the October *Lancet* that he examined his patients under a double fold of a large dark-coloured Paisley shawl. In that case, Simpson replied, it was no wonder that he was inclined to "impale" an organ and have difficulty handling the new instruments. Other writers took sides and Simpson's instruments were defended. One letter reads,

Isaac Irons, being practically unacquainted with the instrument in question, has been led away under the erroneous impression that the uterus was stuck on a piece of metal, something like the hat on his own head; but the truth is, it only requires a careful consideration of the instruments, with due reference to the axis of the womb in situ, soon to satisfy an unprejudiced mind that the term *impaler*, saying nothing about its fearful adjunct, infernal, is a very *unjustifiable* appellation.

If it were not for the spirit so sadly displayed between these two champions respectively of the old and new systems of handling the opposite sex, tending, perhaps not unnaturally, to draw the unfavourable notice of the profession on those appearing to concern themselves in it, I should be tempted to bring forward many other reasons for believing that this invention of Dr. Simpson's which we have frequent opportunities of testing at the hospital, is anything save diabolical contrivances.

> I remain, Sir, your obedient servant,
>> Henry Savage, M.D.,
>> Physician to the Hospital for Women,
>> Orchard Street.

Gloucester Place, Portman-square,
October 1851.

Isaac Irons' attack was unwarranted. On other counts, however, some of Simpson's treatments have been proved wrong. His method of handling the situation when the placenta lay in front of the child has been blamed by current obstetricians as "resulting in a set-back of twenty years in the understanding of haemorrhage and placenta praevia". Simpson believed that the bleeding came from the placenta which should therefore be removed. In fact it came from the severed uterine vessels, and it was not until 1893 that his assistant, Matthews Duncan, came to appreciate this. Irons was quite unjustified in his accusation that Simpson rushed into the operation of Caesarian section: according to the records of the Edinburgh Maternity Hospital, and those of his assistants, Simpson performed the operation very seldom. In his lecture on the subject to his students, he points out that out of 52 Caesarian operations in Britain in the early part of the century, 39 mothers had died, and all the babies. He quoted to his students the case of "Dr Ryan who operated on a fish wife in 1832, who sat up in bed and ate $1\frac{1}{2}$ bushels of cockles on the 3rd day" but this was the exception. Simpson had suggested that Britain's appalling death rate was perhaps due to the fact that the operation was considered "a last resort" whereas, on the Continent, doctors operated before the mother was at her last gasp and with more reserve to cope with the shock of the operation.

Simpson's scientific mind had already dealt with homoepathy. For the same reasons, he could not accept either mesmerism or telepathy, which were now in vogue. In 1851 a public demonstration was held in Edinburgh by a leading exponent. His medium daughter claimed to be able to "divine" the contents of a box in which the audience were invited to place "secrets and sealed papers". Simpson pushed forward from the back of the crowded church hall, along with his friend, the theologian Dr Guthrie. They challenged the medium to state what they had placed in the box. The medium said "money". The box was opened and it was found that Simpson had put in some millet seed, along with a slip of paper on which he had written the word "humbug". The audience was delighted!

Simpson was a believer, however, in the subject of "mind over matter". He wrote a great deal on "spurious pregnancy", in which the patient is quite convinced that she is pregnant, and even exhibits the physical signs that she knows of, such as increased girth. He pointed out that "chloroform is very useful in demonstrating that this is, in fact, just gas". He put forward the idea too, that fear and "mental anguish" could affect the uterine contractions in childbirth, and suggested that this could be overcome by explaining to the patient what was happening and how she could help, and encouraging her to relax by breathing deeply, pre-empting the natural childbirth cult by eighty years.

The *Lancet* had allowed Simpson the last say in the Irons affair, but as usual he complained that the journal took far too long to publish his communications. The answer was to go into the business himself. He became the "proprieter and conductor" of the monthly *Journal of Medical Sciences* and so removed the difficulty of waiting for publication of his own papers.

Simpson was no longer in need of the money from his published works. His pockets were full of the stuff, he wrote to his
sister, sending her £100 in one pound notes. He had two
assistants at this time to help in his practice, who earned £40 a
year. His maids earned 30/– a month and the butler £2.
52 Queen Street was redecorated at this time, and the bill for
the entire house came to £5 17s. 5d.

Dr Channing, the exponent of ether in childbirth in the
States recorded in a letter to Boston, after staying for several
weeks at Queen Street, that,

> Simpson receives a great deal of money, I have heard. But
> he seems wholly regardless of money . . . He is paid at the
> visit or consultation, which saves him from one of the most
> inconvenient offices, charging and collecting fees. We feel
> both the inconvenience and loss in America. I have seen
> fees paid him. It is when the patient is leaving him, and by
> offering the hand for farewell the fee is deposited in his. I
> really think that if he were subjected to our system he would
> get no money at all! "At night," said a patient of his whom
> he sent to me when she came to America "his pockets are
> emptied by his man. He knows nothing of their contents
> before, and is not particularly interested after". I have seen
> him press the guinea, for that it usually is, back into the hand
> of the patient with a "naw, naw, away with ye". The family
> eats choice game or salmon at every meal and finest honey
> and duck eggs, all gifts. This morning before anyone else was
> up I went below for my spectacles. On the sideboard was a
> basket of fine peaches . . . I could fill pages with a list of such
> offerings as are daily poured in. . . . He himself eats little and
> as if almost unconscious of the function.

Channing was impressed too that money could not "buy"
better treatment. His letter continues, "here are the poor and
the rich together with no other distinction than such as will best
accommodate both. And I can say, from a long and wide observation, that there is no difference in their treatment. We spent
as long in the cold cheerlessness with a woman who lay on the
stone floor as in the boudoir of the Duchess".

Simpson enjoyed having money and was always prepared to

hand it out. A Dr Edward Murphy wrote from London imploring Simpson to lend him £100, or at least £50 until some midwifery fees came in, otherwise he "would be in the hands of the Jews". Simpson sent him £200 by return.

The Grindlay family and their sea-captain friends found Simpson ready to listen to many a hare-brained scheme, and prepared to finance any that inspired his enthusiasm. He was talked into speculating in shipping guano from the New Hebrides to Queenstown paying £4,500 for the *Araminta*, the ship that was to carry it; he paid £600 to an Irishman to distil oil from Irish peat, and was persuaded to buy land in Trinidad.

In 1851 Simpson's brother-in-law, Robert Grindlay, asked him to put up £2,000 for the "good ship *Nepaul*". Young Grindlay wrote, "I can hardly believe we have got such a bargain—at least £700 under market price. She should clear £2,000 the first 12 months." The *Nepaul* was to sail under Captain Petrie and her first voyage was from Bahia via Trieste, to the Clyde. By 1858 Simpson and the Grindlays owned between them the 900-ton *British Queen* and the *Falkland* as well as the *Araminta*. The Grindlay shares were actually paid for by Jessie. In 1858 her interest on the loans, plus the balance on the ships, was £3,966 11s. 5d.

The Grindlays seemed free to spend Simpson's money. Robert wrote to Jessie in 1856 asking for another loan of £2,000 and then informed Simpson four days later.

Dear Doctor,
    I have today bought the "Kate Kearney" 349 tons, 2 years old coppered last year, for £2,800—amazingly cheap. I have offered a share of her to no one until I hear from you as if you join us we can take her, third to my mother, third to you and third for us. If you do not like the spec do not let me persuade you. I can easily get others to join. Although I would prefer keeping such a bargain in the family. Thank Jessie for her money in notes.
                                Yours affectionately,
                                R. Grindlay.
Letters from the Nepaul today. There had been two heavy gales off Valparieso but she was safe. Only a for'ard mast broke.

A letter from Jessie to her brother at this time asks if he could find a job on one of the ships for a "certain young lad of 12".

Although inundated with young Scotsmen looking for situations, Walter Grindlay agreed to take this lad on as a ship's carpenter's apprentice at £10 a year. The boy would have to show himself early in the morning, 4.00 or 5.00 a.m. but would be compensated by getting off as soon as 6.00 in the evening. Jessie had been paying £12 three times a year for the upkeep of this boy since 1845.

Jessie was not the only one in Queen Street paying for the upkeep of a child. In May 1852 Simpson gave a baby boy into the care of a Mary Quinton. Simpson told her that this baby was the child of a "lady of high birth" and gave Mrs Quinton £5 for its upkeep and also paid her an additional £2. 10s. od. for a wet nurse for the child for the first half year. Simpson kept in close touch with the child, paying Mrs Quinton a series of cheques that rose from £5 to £25 twice a year and also employed her husband as a secretary. He was an Oxford graduate, and served as an amanuensis. All went well until the Quintons got into financial straits. In 1854 they had taken on a house in Trinity near Viewbank, furnished it on borrowed money, and intended filling it with students to pay the bills. However, no boarders "of a suitable quality" could be found and the creditors were demanding that debts must be met. Jessie Simpson was accustomed to giving Quinton, as her husband's secretary, sums of money to pay her household bills and these he used to meet his own committments. He now asked Simpson for cash to pay the same bills, stole from the butler and borrowed from the medical assistants. One of these, Dr Drummond, went to Simpson and pointed out the situation. Up to his neck in trouble and realising he was now found out, Quinton hid in the attic of his house at Trinity while warrants were issued for his appearance in the debtors' court and his creditors beat on the door.

Mrs Quinton turned to Simpson, begging him to help. Her letter was long and rambling, and unfolded the sordid story of her ineffectual bounder husband. She ends, "let me implore you to save us and your child from this great calamity". Simpson replied that he had had enough of Quinton. Another pleading letter followed containing the suggestion that Simpson was in debt to the Quintons and not the other way around. Simpson answered this by driving to Trinity and giving Quinton £5 and suggesting he use it to flee the town .

Taking this advice, the Quintons absconded to Notting Hill, London, and now they resorted to blackmail. Unless £52 was despatched at once, they threatened to "seek out the mother's address from Professor Syme and disclose all!" For a while Simpson ignored the correspondence, but when the Quintons openly accused him of being the father of the child, he rose to the bait. He flatly denied it, but also refused absolutely to name the parents.

The Quintons were determined to stir up trouble. They wrote to numerous leading Edinburgh figures, then turned to the theologian Dr Guthrie, and demanded that he "see justice done to one who calls himself a Christian".

Simpson replied to the approaches of Dr Guthrie in writing, and sent a copy of his letter to the editors of the two daily papers. As a mirror of the times in dealing with such a situation, perhaps it is worthy of our consideration.

Dear Sir,
    Some time ago you asked the name of the parents of the child whom Mrs Quinton took home some years ago—under the sole condition that he should not be taken back from her by the parents and that he should be entirely surrendered over to her. It is unnecessary, I believe, to state to you that I would trangress most grossly the principles of professinal honour if I complied with such a request. The secret could do no good to Mrs Quinton or the child—as the mother is in poverty and dependence. . . . She may find the parentage of the child from other quarters, if she thinks fit, but she cannot possibly hope to extract the information from me.
    But as you have written on the matter I venture to trouble you with it in another light. Mrs Quinton has written to Professor Syme on the matter. Mr Syme and I are not friends not even on speaking terms, but he has informed Mrs Quinton that he called me to see the mother a few days before the child was born—she having come a long distance to be under the professional care of Mr Syme for supposed tumour. After the child was born I had to make arrange-

G

ments for it being given out to nurse and was thus led into some considerable expense on the matter.

I have heard from a variety of quarters that Mrs Quinton has behaved in the matter in a way which either you must get her to rectify thoroughly at once, or I shall deem it my duty to hand the subject to my lawyers. Mrs Quinton has stated that I am the father of the child. I demand that she forthwith contradict this indelicate suggestion. She well knows who the father is. Out of compassion I refrained many years ago from allowing a most painful prosecution from being instituted against a person in whom she was deeply interested. She is a villainous wicked woman. I expect her to furnish an apology to me.

Yours sincerely,

J. Y. Simpson

The columns of the *Scotsman* seemed entirely given over to the letters to or from J. Y. Simpson in 1852, for it was not long before, another controversy flared, this time involving his usually benign neighbour, Dr Miller.

Mrs Johnstone, a doctor's wife who lived at 34 Queen Street, had died. Simpson had attended her first, then Miller had operated. The surgeon said the patient's death resulted from "peritoneal infection". Simpson did not agree. He felt that she had died from "over bleeding" and that the haemorrhage had been caused by the surgeon cutting an artery by mistake. Miller was the first into print, publishing an attack on Simpson, blaming him for the patient's death.

Other members of the medical profession quickly joined the fray—those jealous of Simpson's social contacts and reputation backing up Miller and decrying Simpson's negligence, and those who felt that surgeons were becoming too important siding with Simpson. Even the bereaved husband, on the very day of his wife's funeral, was forced to state his opinion of the two medical men. He accepted that it was the hand of the Almighty, and not that either doctor had killed his wife. The *Lancet*, having just recovered from the Isaac Irons affair, printed apprehensively "are we now to have a 'Simpson versus Miller' or a 'Miller versus Simpson' out of the latest Edinburgh Quarrel?" And another medical journal pointed out that 'A'

medical attendant put in the position of Miller ought to receive
the sympathy and not the reproach of his brother practitioners"
and that it considered the conduct of "our Edinburgh Fellows
as most undignified and unprofessional".

Simpson was furious that he was the one accused of negligence. He always had to prove that he was right and the other
side most definitely wrong. He now turned detective. Poor Mrs
Johnstone's mattress was retrieved from the laundry; the
position of the blood that saturated it, noted; and the conclusion drawn that only a massive haemorrhage could have
caused so much to flow, and that this was not consistent with a
gentle cupping to treat a pelvic inflammation.

Most leading medical men in Edinburgh belonged to the
Aescalopian Club, and after suffering two months of constant
wrangling between the two doctors, the members decided that
they must use their influence to bring the matter to an end. On
the 17 May 1852 they held a meeting of every member of the
club except Simpson and Miller. They drew up a document
stating that they found

> great disapproval of the conduct pursued by both Drs
> Simpson and Miller. And considering that thereby the
> character of the Medical profession had been greatly injured
> and the peace and harmony of the Club been seriously dis-
> turbed and interrupted, the Meeting resolve,—(without
> expressing their opinion as to the relative amount of blame
> imputable to each of the two members referred to),—that a
> copy of this resolution be sent to both, together with a
> request, that they will take the earliest opportunity of
> expressing their regret for the injury done to the profession,
> and of offering such reparation to the Club as shall be
> satisfactory to the members.

A Swedish doctor, Magnus Ritzius, was staying at 52 Queen
Street as the argument ground to a halt. When he left for
Dublin, he persuaded Simpson to make a sudden decision to go
too. Jessie had just given birth to another boy, Alexander
Magnus, but Simpson's assistants and his influential friend,
Robert Christison, hustled him out of the town on the Glasgow
train in time to catch the steamer across to Ireland.

CHAPTER X

Maturity

SIMPSON HAD LAST been to Dublin in September 1839, just before applying for the Midwifery Chair. He loved the vitality of the Irish capital. He rushed about, infuriating his host, Dr Churchill, at 137 St Stephens Green, by, as Churchill remarked, "scampering hither and thither and disappearing while we pause for breath". Dublin was a Georgian city, divided by the meandering Liffey. The streets and squares compared favourably with Edinburgh's Charlotte Square and Simpson's own Queen Street, but he felt that Edinburgh had nothing as fine as the Dublin Post Office with its six fluted ionic columns, or the "chaste classical colonnades of the Bank of Ireland, set opposite the handsome front of Trinity". He enjoyed meandering through the thronged Grafton Street, listening to the people "talking their begorrahs and full of the blarney". He was struck with the number of carriages and the dozens of jaunting-cars so characteristic of the country. The horses drawing them were better than those to be seen in Edinburgh, and there was far more evidence of wealth. Servants wore gaudy liveries, and there seemed to be more gentlemen in tall hats and coloured frock coats, and ladies in splendid bonnets and flowing rich silk skirts. "Oh, would we had their ostentation," wrote Simpson. "Our life is grey, grey . . . We Scots need rounding off by some Irish song and dance and a little of their joy of life and lightness of tongue."

But Simpson was well aware of the other side of the coin. Sitting on the grand well-scrubbed steps of Dr Churchill's home he would find a ragged woman, huddled in a black fringed shawl; and in order to reach Dr Churchill's magnificent carriage, he once had to step over six wide-eyed, mournful, bare-footed children. There was no work to be had, and beggars wandered about the streets in rags, or lay on the pavement with newspapers as their only protection from the

elements. The London ones were printed on thicker paper than
the local, and were therefore prized for the extra insulation
from the damp, raw cold. Simpson wanted to know where the
poor lived, and so Dr Churchill reluctantly took him to the
"Liberties and back lanes". The indescribable squalor and
wretchedness of the hovels made Edinburgh's teeming Old
Town seem quite respectable. When Simpson insisted on
stopping the carriage for a closer look, eleven ragged urchins
ran up, pulled off the horses' sack of oats, and fought each other
off with one arm while cramming a handful of fodder down
their own throats with the other.

Simpson's archaeological friend, the oculist William Wilde,
took Simpson to a meeting of the Royal Irish Academy where
he met and talked about his new telescope with William Rowan
Hamilton. Hamilton had such a brilliant mind that he had been
elected Professor of Astronomy at Trinity while still an undergraduate. Simpson also met George Petrie, leader of the
antiquarian group in Ireland, who took him to see a Bronze
Age crannog that he had discovered in a lake. The foundations
had been made by heaping stones and earth in a wickerwork
raft until it sank under the weight. More stones and earth were
heaped on until an island rose out of the water. This particular
crannog of Lagore was more complicated than usual, with great
oak beams accurately cemented and nailed together. It was
divided into compartments which contained vast quantities
of bones. Petrie angrily told Simpson that the landlord of the
area, who lived in London, had recently sold 150 cartloads of
bone from the inside of the ancient building, to be used as
manure in Scotland.

Cock fighting and bull baiting could be seen in the streets of
Dublin and Simpson joined a noisy crowd surrounding two
prize fighters, who boxed with bare fists for unlimited rounds.
Dublin's great maternity hospital, the Rotunda, had much to
interest Simpson, but it is interesting to note that he makes no
mention of his old rival, the distinguished Evory Kennedy. The
Rotunda was remarkable in having a special unit for gynaecological complaints, as well as a separate ward for women
actually in labour, and another for women stricken with
puerperal fever, whereas Edinburgh still had no segregation.
Simpson, however, had only one quick dart round the hospital,

before joining Wilde on an expedition over the bogs to see one of his cromlech tombs. Grovelling around in the dark on the site, Simpson put his fingers on a coin. He blew off the dust, then carefully wrapped it up in a crumpled five pound note that he drew out of his pocket. He explained to Wilde that this was to prevent "his man" throwing away the treasured find when he went through his master's pockets, as he always did, at the end of the day.

When Simpson returned to Edinburgh in August of 1853 he was delighted to hear that he had been elected a Foreign Associate of the Academy of Medicine of Paris. This was a highly regarded honour throughout Europe and America. However, the circumstances of Simpson's election caused a stir unparalleled in the history of the Académie de Médecine.

The custom from time immemorial had been for a commission made up of four of the most important and established members to draw up a selected list of prepared names, which the Academy always accepted without comment. On this occasion the list contained seven names of eminent medical men: Baffalino of Florence, Retzius of Stockholm, Ribero of Turin, Warren of Boston, Mott of New York, Wleninch of Brussels, and Grandet of Lisbon, with a supplementary list consisting of Owen, Faraday, and Bright of London.

A leading Paris newspaper reported the critical meeting when the Academy met to elect the new members.

The absence of a name so eminent as Dr Simpson's created the greatest murmur of astonishment and discontent among the more enlightened members of the Academy, and several of them, at the head of whom was Dr Velpeau rose to exclaim against the awkward bévue of which the commission had been guilty. A secret compact was immediately formed and a formal protest agreed upon which, duly signed and sealed was laid upon the President's bureau.

However, the Academy had a rule that demonstrations of free thinking were forbidden, and so the President discarded the protest with scorn. The meeting continued as if nothing had happened and the first six names were duly endorsed; but when the seventh was read out, the members rose to their feet with one accord, waving their arms, shouting "Simpson, Simpson".

Calls of order were completely ignored and the uproar continued. Leaving their seats, the crowd in the body of the hall surged forward around the President's dais and thumped on his desk. In the face of this show, the office bearers capitulated, and Simpson's name was accepted.

As the Paris papers reported, "The event has caused an immense sensation among the medical profession as being totally without example, and already there are pamphlets of all colours, articles and appeals, flying about in all directions . . . the defence of the omission has given birth to the most angry controversy on either side." The speeches made on the occasion gave rise to a display of wit which reflects honour on both parties, while the President himself declared that "although it had hitherto been considered that the greatest honour which the Académie could confer upon a foreign colleague was that of electing him amongst its members, it had remained for Dr Simpson to prove that a greater honour yet existed, that of being chosen in spite of the will of the Académie itself".

In Scotland there were more serious events to think about: in the autumn of 1853 the main topic of conversation in Edinburgh was "the cholera". It was spreading like fingers of cancer through the closes of the Old Town, but, thank Heaven, it hadn't dared to creep down the Mound into the cloistered New. The reaction of the people living in the New Town was rather similar to that demonstrated in medieval days. They would try anything to keep the evil spirits of the disease away. Drinks of herbs and grass were sipped in the drawing rooms, and silken scarves wrapped round the face were considered safer than the customary Paisley shawls. Whiffs of chloroform were declared a help during a carriage journey through the infected air of the city.

As the doctors did not seem to be able to cope with the situation, the people turned to the Church. The Free Church Presbytery took the initiative and on 5 October moved that "the community should be called upon to recognise the hand of God in the visitation". The Moderator of the Established Church. He wrote to the Home Secretary, Palmerston, asking that the Queen declare "a National Day of Prayer and Fast".

Palmerston, however, considered the request "unsuitable" and turned it down. His opinion was that the doctors were at fault, and not God. Negligence caused cholera, he believed, and a few prayers could not make up for a lack of drains. As he stated in his reply to the Moderator, written by Henry Fitzroy:

The best course which the people of this country can pursue to deserve that further progress of the cholera should be stayed, will be to employ the interval that will elapse between the present time and the beginning of next spring in planning and executing measures by which those portions of their towns and cities which are inhabited by the poorest classes, and which from the nature of things, must most need purification and improvement, and be freed from those causes and sources of contagion, which, if allowed to remain, will infallibly breed pestilence, and be fruitful in death in spite of all the prayers and fastings of a united but inactive nation. When man has done his utmost for his own safety, then is the time to invoke the blessing of Heaven to give effect to his exertions.

This letter was read at a mass meeting of the Presbytery of the Church of Scotland. Most of those present took umbrage at this reply from the Home Secretary, and decided to go ahead and have a fast-day of their own. But, one, a friend of Simpson's, Dr Cook, pointed out that while much had been done for the comfort of the rich and for the improvement of their dwellings, little in fact had been done for the poor. "The streets had been watered," he said, "in the more wealthy districts of town in forgetfulness that while doing so, they were hemming the poorer classes into spaces which were not fit for human beings to occupy."

Simpson was taking more and more interest in the affairs of the church. His first positive action in its behalf was when on a visit to Sandy, his brother told him that the Bathgate Free Church was filled with a rabble of dissenters who would not go away until the local ministers appeared, but that he had not the courage to face them. "Turn the lights off," suggested Simpson. Sure enough, the crowd dispersed rather than sit in the cold, dark, cheerless church.

To revert to the cholera in Edinburgh, the Ministers got their fast-day, but moral victory seems to be with Palmerston, backed up by the *Scotsman* and a very few doctors, including Simpson and Cook. In the editorial for 9 November, the *Scotsman* had criticised fast-days on the grounds that they were days of jollification rather than of humiliation. Then on the morning following the fast the paper noted that "a large measure of discontent at the procedure of the Synods exists among all classes, and there is a pretty universal belief that this will be among the last of the 'Fast Days' of this species, and certainly the last that will not meet with an open and pretty general resistance". A few years later administration of fast-days was handed over by the churches to the Town Council for regulation as statutory holidays, and the ministers' extraordinary method of dealing with emergencies gradually died out.

Slowly, too, the cholera outbreak petered out. The dead were duly buried on free land at the top of the Meadows, and the ships in the Firth of Forth that had housed the infected patients returned to their normal business of carrying cargo between Britain and the West Indies. The Grindlay family declared that they had lost "close on £2,000 by having two ships tied up in the Firth", in spite of the Town Council paying them a hiring fee for boarding the sick. Some people had made money out of the epidemic, however: the Newhaven fishermen had made considerable profits by ferrying illicit visitors out to the ships, and by rescuing indignant invalids who considered they were far better off in their own home than aboard the vessels. One evening Simpson found four of these cholera victims hiding in his lilac bushes at Viewbank.

"Infection" was in everyone's thoughts, particularly those of the Royal College of Physicians. Perhaps because of his ailing, and adored daughter Jessie, with her ravishing auburn hair, Simpson's mind at the moment was more occupied with the subject of tuberculosis than cholera. He was concerned with the fact that, as he pointed out in the *Edinburgh Journal of Medical Sciences*, 70,000 people died in Great Britain every year of pulmonary tuberculosis. That worked out at 200 lives a day, 8 every hour, about a life every ten minutes. All treatments so far had been unsuccessful. Visiting the Border town of Galashiels, Simpson had noticed that the people seemed exceptionally healthy, showing none of the ghastly sores that accompanied tuberculosis. This was particularly true of those working in the woollen mills. During the process of weaving, the wool was laced with oil to replace the lanoline lost during the dyeing process. As a result, the weavers were often covered in oil themselves; Simpson now suggested that this was the reason that they never suffered from outbreaks of tuberculosis scrofula on their skin. He immediately put his mind to finding out about the health of weavers in other parts of the country. As his correspondence was answered, Simpson discovered from local doctors that the people in weaving areas accepted the fact that woollen mills were healthy places in which to work. Dr McDougall of Galashiels reported that during the twenty years he had been in practice, he could only remember a few deaths by tuberculosis. He remarked that, before the present Factory Bill was passed, children often worked in the mills ten hours a day, but were extraordinarily healthy as a result, and, to quote his letter to Simpson, "I have myself repeatedly recommended parents to send delicate children to the mills as a prophylactic and always with the most satisfactory results. Consumption in fact is unknown here among the weaving class." The evidence was overwhelming: from Hawick, Alloa, Bridge of Allan, Tillicoultry, Kilmarnock, Selkirk and Inverlieithen came the news that puny, ailing children became stout and healthy after a short time in the wool mills; pale emaciated workers from the cotton mills became rosy and fat when transferred to wool weaving. A doctor with forty-five years' experience in Aberdeen claimed to be able to tell after a glance whether a girl worked with wool or cotton, depending on the colour of her cheeks.

Simpson concluded that the oil wiped away the dirt, thus allowing fresh clear air access to the skin. He quoted Pliny: "The human body receives vigour and strength from every kind of oil", and "there are two liquids very grateful to human bodies namely, wines within and oils without". Perhaps Simpson should receive recognition from the cosmetic advertisers of today in their production of cleansing cream, rather than from the dermatologists.

Although this was one of Simpson's less inspired conclusions, it drew his attention to the subject of "oil" which resulted in some interesting work at an archaeological level.

"What is this peculiar substance oil anyway?" he asked himself. Following his usual methods of research he ferreted out the fact that throughout the ages oil had been prized as a medication as well as an asset to beauty. He remembered also that lepers had often anointed themselves with oil hoping so to arrest their devastating disease. When dashing around the British Museum in London, Simpson had noticed a lead ointment jar with a green label reading "Lukion Paramousaiou", Indian Lykium or "oil of the muses". He tracked down other jars in Paris with similar labels. With infinite trouble he identified the contents as being a substance called Ruswut. The clues then led to the Orient, and through extensive correspondence with doctors in India, he found that Ruswut was still used by the native fakir to relieve trachoma, the eye infection endemic in the East. Robert Christison managed to procure some of the substance for Simpson, who then persuaded his friend Wilde to use it on several cases in his eye infirmary in Dublin. To everyone's surprise, it was successful.

The Ruswut was found near the Irawaddy. This fact lead Simpson to discover that another substance, known as "Rangoon petroleum", was to be found in quantity in deep pits on the sandy banks of that river. It looked like lard at ordinary temperatures, but became quite liquid at 90° Fahrenheit.

It so happened that the manufacturers of Simpson's forceps had their forge in Leith Walk; and that when attempting to mass produce his instrument, they ran into trouble when their newly built machinery seized up. The best anti-friction lubricant, at that time, for finer kinds of heavy machinery, was olive oil, but it was extremely expensive. On hearing of their trouble, Simpson had the idea that Rangoon petroleum would do instead. He immediately rushed around to Christison, whom he knew was using the substance for obtaining paraffin by distillation. Simpson suggested that they try out the idea and if successful, they could take out a patent and so make their fortunes.

Christison agreed, but, as he said when remembering the affair later, "I had long ago resolved never to have any concern in patents"; however, Simpson talked him into agreeing to help with the chemistry. Christison then suggested that when Simpson had made his first £100,000 he might present him with the last thousand, in payment for the first specimen of "Simpon's Incomparable Anti-friction Lubricant".

Having decided when the trial was to take place, Christison called at 52 Queen Street to collect his friend. He found that

"Simpson's two reception rooms were, as usual, full of patients, more were seated in the lobby, female faces stared from all the windows in vacant expectancy, and a lady was ringing the doorbell. But the doctor brushed through the crowd to join me, and left them all kicking their heels at their leisure for the next two hours". At the factory in Leith, they found that the machine which marked 100 when arrested by friction without any lubricant, indicated 38 with olive oil, and only 6 with the Rangoon Petroleum. Simpson wrote at once to the Patent Office in London, only to find that one had been taken out for the very same idea a few days before. Undaunted, Simpson turned his attention to cod liver oil and then sperm whale oil. This led him to approach his brother in law, Captain Petrie, asking him to procure some sperm whale oil. The captain replied to the letter of inquiry with an interesting account of life at sea in the immortal days of Moby Dick.

Sea-View,
December 26, 1854.

My Dear Doctor,

I am happy to be able to communicate to you the particulars you desire, respecting the sperm whale.

In the latter part of the year 1831, I embraced the opportunity of carrying out a voyage to the South Seas, for the purpose of procuring sperm oil. Knowing that the sperm whale was difficult and dangerous to capture. I deemed it necessary to adopt some other means of lifting them. I think it was my brother the doctor who suggested to me a trial of prussic acid, if any way could be contrived of introducing the poison into the blood. The plan of doing this was entirely my own invention. I had a convenient and portable hearth and bellows for the purpose of manufacturing suitable harpoons provided on board the ship *Betsy* . . . After having the ship fitted for a South Sea voyage, we left Portsmouth in December of the same year and arrived at Sydney in May 1833, where the *Betsy* was completely fitted with everything necessary for procuring a cargo of sperm oil in the Pacific Ocean. For the purpose of killing whales readily, I had procured a considerable quantity of prussic acid, and with my new harpoon, I hoped to succeed in doing wonders with the Scotch Whaler, or prussic acid ship, as the *Betsy* was called. After being very fortunate among the Solomon Islands and Japanese Seas, I had a fair opportunity of trying my new harpoon. Unfortunately, the bottles of prussic acid being round, resisted the pressure which expected would be sufficient to break them, two being attached to the harpoon. The harpoon being constructed this way, having the usual length of shank with the smaller head sharp and steeled at the lower part. A strong joint was carved on each side for a movable wing four inches long, kept sufficiently off the shank to allow a bottle of prussic acid on each side.

In consequence of not having proper bottles for the purpose, it did not work. I lost the chance of giving my experiment a fair trial. You wished to know how the harpoon acts in catching a whale. It is generally endeavoured as to send in two harpoons for fear of one misgiving, as near the upper part of the back of the fin as possible. If they go no further than the blubber, the harpoon will seldom hold. The region of the heart is usually arrived at, for, if the harpoon can be made to touch the heart, death is certain. The whale blows up a prodiguous quantity of blood, and the greatest danger to the boats is during this death struggle. The largest sperm whale will produce about twelve tons of oil, yielding about 960 pounds, but we only captured one this size. The average is usually 70 barrels. The largest whale we captured had an enormous quantity of sperm in a liquid state. Soon after this, our ship came across some Americans, but the Scotch whaler, *Betsy* of Leith was more than a match for them. The *Betsy* had on board about 20 Scotch youths as part of her crew, who had been accustomed to use the oar at Newhaven, and were always found very powerful and dexterous in its use. The *Betsy* captured a valuable sperm whale in the very face of the American whaler, the captain of which saw one of my harpoons and was so delighted with it, he wished particularly to buy it. I refused for some time until he offered me a barrel of molasses, an article which we were in want of, and he got it.

I am dear Doctor,

Yours sincerely,
P. Petrie.

Simpson's knowledge of such things as sperm whales greatly impressed John Ruskin when he visited Edinburgh in 1853. Simpson and he dined together at the house of the Professor of Natural History, Robert Jameson, and Ruskin wrote in his diary,

> Dr Simpson tells me for the first time in my life the meaning of "Chief Prince of Meschech and Zubal" (Ezekiel xxxix).
> Meschech—Western Russia, a portion of this word still remaining in Moxcow or Moscowa.
> Zubal—Siberia—the word remaining in Zobolski.

The conversation round the dinner table that evening then turned to ghosts and second sight, and Simpson enthralled the party by relating the story of one of his patients who suddenly, in the middle of a dinner party at which he was present, gave a terrible shriek, then fell down in a dead faint behind the table. On coming round, she clutched Simpson in terror and explained that the corpse of an old sweetheart had appeared in front of her. Simpson declared that the only way for her to appreciate that this was pure imagination was for her to look at a genuine dead body. He took her to his dissecting room, and made her lift up the arm of a corpse. The lady then admitted to Simpson that she had several times also seen the dead body of her sister lying at the foot of her bed. Now, however, having compared the touch of a real corpse, she could convince herself that it was fantasy.

Ruskin, the hypochondriac, asked Simpson if he thought he could cure his assorted ailments by suggestion. Simpson replied "very possibly". Simpson had treated Ruskin's wife, Effie Grey, in 1849. He diagnosed "a nervous complaint of long standing", and had suggested that what she needed were a few children to occupy her mind. In 1853 Effie wrote to her mother in Perth, "I have been very fortunate about Simpson. He came to me yesterday, and again today . . . diagnosed tonsilitis, prescribed chloroform pills, and the same for Millais." Millais was the painter with whom Effie fell in love soon after her frustrating marriage with Ruskin. She claimed that Ruskin had never consummated their marriage and was in fact impotent. Simpson's evidence was used on Effie's behalf when the question was brought into the court in 18⬛. Eventually, Effie had several children by Millais, perhaps proving her point! Several of the University Chairs change occupants, during 1853 and early '54, and Simpson was involved on each occasion. He canvassed for his candidate by letters to such influential friends as the Duke of Argyll, Lords Balfour and Elcho. Simpson wanted to bring the American naturalist Agassiz to Edinburgh, to fill the Chair of Natural History, but the American's views were considered too advanced and likely to lead to trouble with the theologians, and so much to Simpson's regret he was not appointed.

Simpson had been elected President of the Medico Chirurgical Society in 1853. His address on taking the Chair was "On the Modern Advancement of Physic". The paper was an assessment of the point which medicine had reached by the mid-century, and summed up the knowledge gleaned during the last fifty years. Simpson began his address by stressing the importance of such societies as the Medico Chirurgical as a stimulant to original thought. The action of mind on mind; one idea leading to another; the members infecting each other with a kind of intellectual contagion.

He mentioned Watt's rediscovery of the steam engine and the development of the steamboat, railway, and the electric telegraph; then there was the telescope which, together with the calculus of the mathematician, had recently unfolded the solar system; and now there was the brilliant use of light in the discovery of the photograph. But medicine, Simpson pointed out, had been keeping step with these advances. Chemistry had been revolutionised with the atomic theory, and anatomy had seen the birth of embryology and the idea that tissues consisted of nucleated cells.

It was in the new science of pathology, Simpson continued that there had been the greatest advancement on the medical front. Pathology had thrown a new light on disease, it separated "inflammation of the lungs" into pleurisy, pneumonia, bronchitis; it segregated tumours into various types and isolated diseases of the heart. It was now possible to trace and understand the course of inflammation, tuberculosis, and cancerous growths. The microscope was the magic eye with which the pathologist could predict the malignant course of a tumour or diagnose diseases of the organs and blood.

The stethoscope had been another great step in physical diagnosis, and the previous thirty years had also added many new drugs to the Pharmacopoeia, such as iodine, hydrocyanide, and cod liver oil. But, predicted Simpson, soon medicines would be administered by quicker and more efficient routes than through the stomach; by inhalation and by injection. Drugs affect the system with far greater rapidity this way, he stated, than when swallowed in the traditional manner.

Surgery's greatest advance was the silken thread, now used to arrest haemorrhage. This meant the end of the terrifying days of the searing irons. (This silken ligature had one more step to go—that of joining the lips of a wound without causing suppurative inflammation.) Altogether, Simpson remarked surgery demanded far less heroism. Bones were excised where whole limbs had once been cut off, and aneurysms compressed instead of being laid open amid a fountain of blood and spew of guts. The surgeon now boasted of the cases on which he did not operate, such as the cure of hydrocele by injection, instead of incision. It was also only during the last thirty years that the surgeon had directed his attention to the cause of death after an operation. He now knew that it was not haemorrhage, but blood poisoning that killed the patient; it remained to find some direct antidote to the poison as it circulated in the blood. Also, of course, Simpson added, the surgeon now had the power of wrapping the patient in a dreamless sleep, thus realising the enchantment of the Arabian Nights and the spells of bygone days.

In practical medicine the half-century had seen the replacement of dungeons for the insane by clean asylums, the end of scurvy in the fleet, the treatment of goitre, and the new-fangled idea that prevention was better than a cure. The hygiene and management of children and infants was now considered a subject on its own. One hundred years ago, stated Simpson, 60 out of every 100 children born in London, died before reaching the age of five. Now, the mortality rate had diminished to 30 per cent. Public Health had come into being and it was now appreciated that communities needed sufficient fresh air, water and drainage, and adequate refuse collection. But, Simpson shouted at his complacent audience, only a fraction of this promising work had been accomplished, and the expectancy of life in a crowded city was still only a third of that in a rural community.

The greatest victory of medicine over disease during the last fifty years was, of course, vaccination; and Simpson put the name of Jenner at the top of the list. Military science had invented new and dreadful machinery, but, Simpson remarked, "the millions of money expended in the vast military stores at Woolwich and Cherbourg lack the ability to destroy human life to any such degree as one drop of despised cow pox matter . . . has the ability to save it".

However, according to the Registrar General, there were still 50,000 deaths a year from consumption; 30,000 from pneumonia; 20,000 from typhus and scarlet fever; and, more horrifying, 3,000 mothers still perished in childbirth. So there was much to be done. How about inoculation against the whole class of non-recurrent disease, such as whooping cough, measles, and scarlet fever?

Simpson ended his address with a pledge to promote kindliness and good fellowship among the members of the society! He would encourage debate, he promised the audience, but nothing was to be said that could hurt the feelings of any of the profession, absent or present, and while he was in the chair, the Society would cultivate the heart as well as the mind. The audience was delighted to hear this last remark, and was prepared to believe that Simpson had turned over a new leaf.

The Society flourished under Simpson and became a meeting place for Continental and American visitors to the city. The main topic of conversation among doctors at this time was "infection". Every pregnant woman and most obstetricians had their minds on the subject of puerperal fever. As Simpson pointed out in his address, more women died of it now than in the days before the care and attention available in the maternity wards and Lying-in Hospitals now spread over the country. He also considered that puerperal fever was the same disease as surgical fever, and that death resulted in both cases for the same reasons. Since 1840, Simpson had taught his students that,

There exists, I believe, a series of facts amply sufficient to prove that patients during labour have been inoculated with the material capable of exciting puerperal fever. This material is inoculated into the dilated and abraded lining of the maternal passages . . . by the fingers of the attendant. That thus in transferring from patient to another, the fingers act like the ivory points formerly used by the early vaccinators.

Simpson was adamant that the fever was passed not from one patient to another, but through the medium of a third person who was usually the medical attendant or the nurse. He bore this out by studying the cases attended by numerous doctors, finding that the incidence of the disease was often limited to a single practitioner in a town. Simpson quoted a Dr Hill of Leuchars, who reported that a carpenter in his area had injured his hand while lifting a corpse into a coffin. The wound became infected and a severe attack of septicaemia set in. Subsequently, his wife had a similar attack. Their daughter living with them and seven months pregnant, then became ill, and a few days later gave birth to a dead child. The girl herself died within twenty-four hours with the symptoms of puerperal fever. On his road home from visiting this patient Dr Hill was called to a case in labour and this woman also was attacked by the fever and died. Simpson summed up the question by remarking, "We cannot fancy that this 'something' that is carried from one woman to the next consists of ought else than some form of that virus to which pathologists give the name of contagion."

This was not an original thought. In 1773 Charles White of Manchester, an enlightened man midwife had published a paper recommending "antiseptic injections" into the uterus, and insisting on strict cleanliness and ventilation. Then in 1795 Alexander Gordon of Aberdeen published a *Treatise on the epidemic Puerperal Fever of Aberdeen* in which he advised nurses and doctors who had attended cases of the fever to wash their hands and fumigate their clothes, and was the first writer to show clearly the infectious nature of the fever and the way in which it was spread. He considered that fresh air and cleanliness were not enough for the "destruction of contagion" and was a great believer in fire and smoke.

At the turn of the century almost all the knowledge on the subject had been accumulated, but it still needed someone with vision to sort it out. By the early 1840s it was accepted practice in Britain in the teaching hospitals to wash hands and burn bed

linen. Dr Rigby of London, Dr Douglas of Dublin, and many
other influential doctors appreciated that the condition was
infectious and could be prevented by cleanliness, but in spite
of this, women were still dying from the disease in areas dotted
all over the country. America then took up the challenge, and
in 1843, Oliver Wendel Holmes, who was a doctor as well as an
author, though not an obstetrician, raised a storm of hostile
argument by his paper, "On the Contagiousness of Puerperal
Fever". He wrote clearly and precisely and was too highly
thought of by the public to be disregarded. But his simple
suggestion of washing hands and changing clothes between
each case was thrown out by the medical establishment as an
insult, in spite of an array of the most convincing evidence. The
same Meigs who considered the pain of childbirth "beneficial"
threw bitter sarcasm at Holmes, and had another dig at Simpson by pointing out that the Edinburgh doctor had puerperal
patients in spite of having clean hands. Or were they clean?

Holmes silenced his critics by his literary rather than his
medical talents. Having listed the causes of the fever, he called
the doctor who disregarded them a criminal, and, carried on,

> . . . I call up the memory of these irreparable errors and
> wrongs. No tongue can tell the heartbreaking calamity they
> have caused; they have closed the eyes just opened upon a
> new world of love, and happiness; they have bowed the
> strength of manhood into dust; they have cast the helplessness
> of infancy into the strangers arms, or bequeathed it, with less
> cruelty, the death of its dying parent. There is no tone deep
> enough for regret, and no voice loud enough for warning . . .
> God forbid that any member of the profession to which she
> trusts her life, doubly precious at that eventful period, should
> hazard it negligently, inadvisably, or selfishly.

The battle against puerperal fever was won by Ignaz Semmel
weis, a Hungarian working in Vienna. The Lying-in Department of the Vienna General Hospital was divided into two
clinics, one for the teaching of medical students, and the other
for instructing the midwives. Semmelweis soon noticed that the
death-rate in the students' clinic was far higher than the one in
which the midwives were taught. The patients had also noticed

this, and pleaded to be treated by the midwives. They would scream and weep at the door of the students clinic, and many babies were born in the street. During one year, 460 women died in the one clinic and only 105 in the other. Semmelweis' superiors accepted this fact, but he asked why? He appreciated that the problem was infection, but he had somehow to prove his point. He considered the situations in both clinics and spent four years eliminating the differences. Then in 1846 a professor cut his finger during a post mortem and died. Suddenly, Semmelweis realised that the professor's symptoms were exactly the same as those of the woman he had examined who had died from puerperal fever. This led him to conclude that the medical students must be carrying the infectious material from the dead bodies in the dissecting-room, to the women in labour in the wards.

In May 1847 Semmelweis annoyed his students by insisting that they scrubbed their hands in a solution of chloride of lime before they touched any patient. Immediately the death rate fell from 11·4 per cent in 1846 to 3·8 per cent by the end of 1847. Semmelweis then made known his positive proof of the way in which puerperal fever was caused. The first published account of his doctrine appeared in the December issue of the *Journal of Medical Sciences of Vienna* in 1847 written by the editor, Dr Hebra. The jigsaw was complete. Semmelweis realised that he himself had been responsible on many occasions for carrying the infection from a dead body to a healthy woman. As he admitted, "Consequently, must I here make my confession that God only knows the number of women whom I have consigned prematurely to the grave". But Semmelweis was no writer, and so his work was only propagated by word of mouth. His results were so little known that when Homes wrote a further paper as late as 1865, the American misquoted his name and referred to him as "Sendersein".

To his surprise, Semmelweis's theory was not accepted. Doctors reacted with scorn and disbelief, and, as we have seen, Simpson himself was not encouraging. He felt that the high incidence of puerperal fever on the Continent was due to the appalling conditions in the wards. A woman in Paris, for instance, would be admitted to hospital and placed in a bed that a corpse was still occupying, and both would end up in the same coffin. The linen and blankets were not changed and not a glimmer of sunlight or breath of fresh air was allowed into the wards.

Simpson wrote to Semmelweis that he "knew for certain that the cause of the high mortality lay only in the unbounded carelessness with which patients are treated". Semmelweis agreed that the criticism of conditions in Vienna was only too just, and reiterated that chloride of lime would combat any casualness in the care of the patient. But Semmelweis was considered by his superiors too young to have made any clever deductions and so he lost his job and had to leave Vienna in 1849.

By 1854 Simpson realised that there was more in Semmelweis's doctrine than he had at first appreciated. The Hungarian was now working at Pesth, and in five years he had reduced mortality among his 200 cases a year to the unheard-of rate of 0·85 per cent. Semmelweis should have published this fantastic proof of the success of his method at this point, but he hated writing and he believed that, as his doctrine was true, it would be spread without anything more than a few letters and occasional lectures by his friends. Simpson, among others, urged him to set down his own principles, and in 1857 he reluctantly agreed, but the manuscript was not finished until August 1861, the book appearing in October. This reluctance to publish resulting in the holding back of pioneering work by fourteen years, has an analogy in our time: the critical observations with regard to penicillin were made in the 1930s but the principle of antibiosis was not made use of until the 40s.

Simpson's part in the eradication of puerperal fever is clouded by the fact that he did not jump to champion Semmelweis in 1847. He made up for this ommission several years later when he did a great deal to propagate the principles of the Hungarian. In 1854 Simpson announced that he had been in error in rejecting Semmelweis's doctrine and soon became one of its most ardent advocates. Dr John Denham, then Master of the Dublin Rotunda, writing in the *Dublin Quarterly Journal of Medical Sciences* in 1862, criticised Simpson who "holds strongly the infectious character of the disease and, I regret to add, makes the doctor bear the sin and disgrace of spreading the disease".

Semmelweis did not live to see the vindication of his theory. In 1863, when forty-three, he started to have fits of depression, and by 1865 he was considered insane. When he arrived at the asylum, a nurse noticed that he had injured his right hand. He had wounded it during his last operation on a puerperal-fever patient. Two days later he was dead from the disease that he had devoted his professional life to preventing.

Ironically, at just this time Joseph Lister was preparing his inspired paper, "On the Antiseptic Principle in Surgery". Young Lister had come to Edinburgh in 1853. It was Simpson's friend, the avuncular William Sharpey, who suggested to Lister that he go to Edinburgh to complete his surgical studies. As we have seen, Sharpey had also been a friend of Syme ever since the time when they had both studied in Paris, and Lister carried a letter of introduction to Syme, and the young man came North for a month. Syme's beautiful daughter Agnes liked the new "dresser" (surgeon's assistant), and walked with him over Arthur's Seat and down to Duddingston Loch. She helped Lister catch frogs among the reeds, and this unromantic pursuit led to their marriage in 1856, and also the publication of his paper, "The Early Stages of Inflammation", which set him off on his life's work.

Meanwhile, Simpson spent New Year's Eve of 1854 with an English guest whom he had invited to 52 Queen Street, Dr Spencer Wells. Spencer Wells was the editor of the *Medical Times and Gazette*, with offices in Soho, and it was in this connection that the two men came together.

In a letter of 9 July 1853, Wells had written to Simpson that his journal would take "every opportunity of advocating your claims upon the Nation in connection with chloroform". In return, Wells asked Simpson to send him some "cases of plastic operation—ruptured perineum, vessico, or recto vaginal fistula . . . I don't want them to pay me, provided they don't put me to any expense."

Simpson had invited Wells to Edinburgh at the end of 1853, to operate on a fistula, but first of all Wells had to survive Hogmanay. Wells published this account of the occasion:

The night was spent with Simpson, Priestly, and others in visiting the prison, whisky shops and low haunts of that city. Next day among S. private hospital work. At night S. entered

into a learned discussion at the Royal Society on some of the
Buddhist opinions and monuments of Asia compared with the
symbols of the ancient Sculptured Standing Stones of Scotland. Afterwards S. drove S.W. to a country house, the scene
of the ball in Waverley, where patients were visited in the
middle of the night, the home and grounds seen by moon-
light, and Edinburgh only reached in the early morning.
That day Mr Wells did his operation in the Edinburgh
Infirmary and returned to London in the evening. S. having
been in bed only two hours all this time—no uncommon
example, it was said, of his marvellous activity and power of
work.

Unfortunately, Wells had to use silk sutures for the operation
in the Edinburgh Infirmary, and not the metal ones that he
preferred, and the operation was not successful. Wells insisted
on strict cleanliness when he operated, without being able to
give a clear reason. He also insisted on silence in the theatre.

The conversation between Simpson and Wells during this
visit must have centred round the War that Wells was to join
in a month's time. The Crimean offensive had broken out the
preceding September. The ill-equipped British troops had
landed on the Peninsula to fight the battle of the Alma. Already
reports of the appalling conditions among the wounded were
filtering home. The medical organisation was non existent, but
thanks to the correspondent of *The Times*, the British public
were well informed, and enthusiastically rallied to the cause of
the wounded. Florence Nightingale began to organise her
nurses for Scutari, and she wrote to Simpson asking for information on the use of chloroform in the field. She also asked
Duncan and Flockhart to supply her with some of the drug free.
They refused, but Simpson bought her enough for 1,000 doses,
and it was duly despatched.

Simpson condemned the war. When presenting his students
for graduation in 1856, he reporoved the politicians who were
behind it. He disapproved strongly of what he called "un-
civilised incitements" to the young men to join the fight and
the "false patriotic" shouts of "Pride, Pomp, and Circumstance
of Glorious War". Lord Cardigan was no hero of his, Simpson
declared, pointing out to the new graduates that the easiest

and surest path to the peerage book was to destroy diligently and successfully as many as possible of their fellow men.

Simpson urged the new graduates not to rush to the Crimea, but to go and fight the crusade for better health all over the habitable globe. "To give ease to the agonized, strength to the weak, health to the sick and sometimes life to the dying." In particular, he asked them to calm the cries of pain and anguish of the women of the world. And, always "to soothe, even when you cannot save".

Despite his disapproval, Simpson was extremely interested in the course of the war, and kept up to date with the news by having a stream of visitors to Queen Street to give him first-hand accounts of the scene. "Do you ken Simpson?" the butler asked a stranger on the doorstep at No. 52. "No, but I've been to the Crimea," was the reply. "Och, weel, you'd best come in then," reluctantly agreed the butler with a sigh.

As the disastrous war ground on, the press looked around for someone to blame. The pointing finger even singled out Simpson, and announced that he was the cause of it all. If it hadn't been for his chloroform, soldiers would never have agreed to the possible agonies of field amputation, the usual treatment for every gunshot wound, and the war would have come to a complete halt for lack of men.

Civilian life in Britain was little affected by the war, and in the summer Simpson spent a very happy week in Ireland, riding across the island from the Giant's Causeway to Cork and from Athlone to Dublin. This was one of the very few trips on which Jessie bestirred herself to accompany her husband. Young Jessie, Simpson's "sunbeam", went too. She and her mother fell out of an Irish gig in the Phoenix Park, but no one was hurt. Simpson loved his daughter's company, and hustled her up round-towers and into old churches, enjoying sharing his enthusiasm and making discoveries together. He wrote to a friend, "Jessie and I did become such tremendous cronies on the road. She was all activity, was one day up at half past five and not in bed till after eleven—pretty well for a young lady of eight years. She rode her horse for six miles at the head of the Killarney Lakes and was rejoiced at 'beating' both her mother and me." The toddler, Magnus Retzius, had been left at home with the older children. He was the image of his father, tubby and square, short legged, with an engaging smile, fat red cheeks, and curly reddish hair. He put his foot in his first birthday cake, much to the amusement of his father. Although he was always in trouble, everyone loved Retzius and his chubby cheeks were well kissed. He was particularly ticklish under his chin, and Simpson's patients reported seeing the little boy stumbling into the waiting room, shrieking with laughter as his father caught up with him and rubbed his hairy whiskers along the child's neck till he was convulsed with giggles.

On his return from Ireland, two assistants announced that it was high time that Simpson's numerous papers were gathered together in book form and suggested that they undertook the job themselves. Simpson was very flattered. He wrote to a friend, Mrs Total, in early 1855,

Drs Priestly and Storer, my two assistants at present, are bringing out an edition of all the sense and nonsense I have ever written on Midwifery. It is their own idea; and Messrs Black are to pay all expenses, and give them £100 for every 1,000 copies sold. I sometimes am allowed to see a proof sheet. It is to be a work, it appears, of 1,200 or 1,400 octavo pages. They have printed last month 500 pages.

This book, *Obstetric Memoirs and Contributions*, was a great success. Within two months of publication, 10,000 copies were sold in the U.S.A. Soon after this, Storer returned to his native America to join the staff of the Boston Lying-in Hospital, which no doubt further increased the circulation. Simpson was relieved to have his assistants handle the book. During the winter of '55 he began to complain of frequent headaches and pain in the side of his chest. He whipped over to Paris in the spring of '56 to see if a short holiday away from his demanding pateints would renew his vitality. His crammed his five-day stay with visits to archaeologists, hospitals and museums.

He returned to Edinburgh in time for the birth of his ninth and last child, a girl, christened Evelyn Blantyre after her godmother. Simpson wrote to a friend in his old jocular style, "A report has been current here for the last thirty hours that there is a new baby upstairs. Walter thinks I must have brought it from France and is terrified it will only speak French. Wee

Jessie says it is a good boy and she will nurse it. Mrs S. is quite
well, and was of course, sound asleep when this little stranger
arrived.

Soon after Eve's birth Simpson made her godmother Lady
Blantyre the child's legal guardian. Simpson was very superstitious. Was this extraordinary step taken because of the pains
in his chest or because he knew his wife to be slipping downhill? Soon after this, a pane of glass was fitted in the door of
Jessie's room so that her actions could be supervised. Eve's
association with Lady Blantyre led her to be a close friend of
Robert Louis Stevenson. The two young people used to skate
together on Duddingston Loch, and Eve enjoyed the company
of the moody, delicate boy. Simpson's son Walter also became a
friend of Stevenson and accompanied him on a tour to Europe.
Later Eve gathered together her recollections into a biography
of Stevenson's Edinburgh days. Eve outlived her eight brothers
and sisters, and is remembered by three of her second cousins
to this day. They recollect her as sparkling and witty, a fine
story teller, an ardent believer in the second sight, as wielding
a lively pen, and a great companion. She never married, so
these talents, that were a mirror of her father's, were not handed
on for this generation to enjoy.

However, to return to 1856, Eve's father made no concessions
to ill health and never let up with his work. He published three
medical papers that summer, and delivered seven addresses to
an assortment of physicians associations. He had a quick tour
of the Lake District and three days on the Isle of Man as well as
answering calls to deliver babies in Perth, Aberdeen and down
the Clyde.

Mr Horace Greeley, the editor of the *New York Tribune*, sent
home this impression of a visit to 52 Queen Street in 1856,

[Simpson] is the index and dictionary of Edinburgh and half
the world beside, and open to everybody that can get
through the crowd forever pressing round for a peep. . . .
Assembled unceremoniously in a moderate sized room with
nothing in common save their wish to meet the host. You find
a company drawn together from every latitude and longitude
social and geographical. . . . At your elbow, the last survivor
of some well known shipwreck is telling his terrible story to

the wife of that Northern Ambassador who is meeting with
the softest of the Scandinavian dialects the strong maritime
Danish of the clever State Secretary opposite. Behind you, a
knot of American Physicians just arrived, are discussing in
their loud voice, the subject of slavery. That lady, with the
fine Greek profile of face and sad grey hair is telling how
Tennyson used to visit the house of her mother and knowing
that they disliked smoke, he used to sit and puff it up the
chimney. . . . You may catch something of yonder violent
discussion between these arrivals from Australia who have
come from the land of gold in search of what gold cannot buy.
You are still learning the last price of provisions in Melbourne
. . . when a carriage in full pace suddenly stops and in a
minute, Dr Simpson enters . . . with a few genial nods, smiles
and shakes of the hand. He begins to dispatch the coffee and
roll put ready for him, and you are impressed with the
womanly softness of the eyes, the amiable play of the mouth
that looked just now stern set and determined, but which is
moving in all manner of ready sympathy or good natural
drollery. Eating, drinking, opening and reading the heap of
letters waiting him, writing a one line response to some
request of friendship, while a brother professor at one ear
propounds a question of University discipline. . . . In ten
minutes the indefatigable Professor is again professorial.
Beckoning some patient he disappears. . . . Meanwhile, news
comes by telegraph that some poor peasant's wife is in the
dangerous stage of some calamity. There are none-knows-
how-many wealthy invalids waiting, but kind heartedness
and delights of a desperate case prevail, and the Doctor is
off across the Forth and will not be back 'till midnight. . . .

The Crimean War was over by mid summer of 1856 and the
French and British Governments could think of other things.
Simpson received a letter from the British Embassy in Paris
announcing that the French Academy of Sciences had awarded
him the Monthyon Prize. The citation read that the presentation was due to Simpson's "most important benefit conferred to
humanity by the introduction of chloroform into Midwifery
and surgical practice". Enclosed were two 1,000 franc notes
plus a handsome gold medal.

King Oscar of Sweden also decided to honour Simpson and presented him with the Royal Order of St Olaf, for "the introduction of chloroform and forcing its acceptance by the medical profession". Spencer Wells, writing in congratulation remarked that it was high time Queen Victoria followed suit.

Simpson and Wells were corresponding at this time on the subject of cancer and its cures, and exhchanging gossip of curers, their fees and their failures. A Dr Fell in London declared that he had a secret ointment that could heal a cancer sore. So Wells, who practised surgery in London in addition to editing the *Medical Times and Gazette* went along to see him, and reported his visit to Simpson. "I fancy he used a chloride of zinc, coloured with Prussian blue and antimony . . . I have seen many of his patients." Fell had confidently stated that his cure was painless, so Wells was particularly interested to note that in fact his patients suffered a great deal. However, as Fell "assured them that they were not and could not be in pain, they seem to believe him, or are afraid of offending him by confessing to pain". Simpson, meanwhile, visited an old woman in Fife, whom his antiquarian friend, Douglas Laing, had told him knew a cure for tumours, which consisted of an ointment that also contained zinc. This eighty-year-old woman lived in a cave, and she mixed the zinc ointment with seaweed. Simpson noted in his letter to Wells that there were two church ministers' wives sitting outside the cave, waiting for treatment from the old crone. He watched while the women applied the ointment to sores on their breasts, but he decided that they were suffering from simple inflammatory ulcerations and not cancer at all.

Before the year was out Simpson had one quick jaunt to Inchcolm. On a November afternoon, when the Forth was absolutely still and a mistiness hung over the water, Simpson borrowed a little yacht and sailed across to the island. Hans Andersen, when dining at Queen Street, had asked Simpson if there was any evidence of Celtic "magic markings" in the ruin on the island that Simpson had recently discovered. This return visit was for the purpose of finding an answer to the Dane's question. This ruin was being used as a pig-sty, but Simpson declared that it was actually a religious hermit's cell, dating from the twelfth century. Simpson pointed this out to the proprietor, the Earl of Moray and the animals were removed and the building repaired by an architect friend of Simpson's, Mr Brash of Cork.

Christison accompanied Simpson on this trip and went off to watch birds while Simpson studied the ruin. Underneath the moss and dirt of ages, Simpson did indeed find some markings scratched on the old stones. He carefully copied them and later compared them to Hans Andersen's diagrams of similar inscriptions found in Denmark. It was dark by the time the two men left the island and they were late for their tea. Hastily swallowing this down, Simpson went straight on to a confinement in the Old Town which kept him for fourteen hours.

During that winter Simpson escaped from Edinburgh for a welcome business trip to Abbotsford where he delivered Sir Walter Scott's first great-grandson. He was called Michael after the wizard, but was, as Simpson reported, "but a very wee, wee wizard himself".

At Christmas a wealthy patient presented Mrs Simpson with a portrait of her husband by Sir John Watson Gordon. The artist apologised for any discrepancies in the portrait, explaining that most of it was from memory, as Simpson hardly ever appeared for a sitting and, when he did, asked questions on such topics as how the WaiAna Indians of Surinam procured their red dye, and the source of vermilion.

When the year's class of forty-three medical students graduated at the end of the Candlemas Term, Simpson was delighted that one of the four most outstanding students was his favourite brother Sandy's son, Alexander.

Simpson took an enthusiastic interest in "Aleck", who later became a distinguished obstetrician in his own right. He was eventually appointed to Simpson's own chair, which he occupied for thirty-five years, resigning in 1905 at the age of seventy. He also brought up his family of six sons and two daughters in 52 Queen Street, and it is only recently that the house has changed hands. Alexander was killed at the age of ninety-one by one of the new-fangled motor cars which zoomed along Queen Street at the awful speed of twenty-five miles per hour. The elderly professor walked straight into its path.

The midwifery chair that Simpson and then Alexander occupied was the oldest in the world. Despite the advances made in the obstetrics field Edinburgh was still unusual in that it considered midwifery as a subject in its own right; many universities felt that a graduate could be an adequate doctor and yet know nothing of obstetrics. In Cambridge midwifery was not mentioned in connection with the final M.B. examination until 1859—preceding Oxford by just one year. Students graduated from a University in Britain, but a licence actually to practice medicine was only granted by one of the Royal Colleges of Physicians or of Surgeons.

As we have seen, Simpson had much to do with the acceptance of midwifery as a respectable branch of medicine; now he became involved with the inception of professionalism in medicine. Until 1858 there were physicians and surgeons and "barber-surgeons" and "apothecaries", all of whom scarcely recognised each other as colleagues. The Royal Colleges had no authority outside their own areas. In the remainder of the country an Edinburgh, Oxford or Cambridge graduate, a President of a Royal College, or the Dean of a medical school, had no more right to practice than the chemist or the village blacksmith who often still hung out his board offering to let blood and draw teeth.

For many years there had been a feeling in medical circles that something must be done about this situation. The general public had no way of distinguishing a qualified practitioner from a quack. It was Syme who took the first concrete step. He published a letter to Lord Palmerston suggesting that the Queen appoint a medical board for regulating the education and practice of doctors in Great Britain and Ireland. He recommended that the board should determine the minimum standards of education necessary before a licence was conferred and publish a register of those who qualified. The board should also be in a position to punish those who assumed false titles.

Palmerston agreed with Syme, and the idea was put out to leading medical men for their views. This created a situation similar to a well-stirred nest of agitated hornets. There were as many opinions as doctors, and tempers began to frey as each tried to stress his personal point. Those of Edinburgh felt particularly concerned, as her Royal Colleges of Physicians and Surgeons were extremely jealous of their position, and were frightened of dilution. They had been going for a very long time, and considered their qualifications for membership of a far higher standard than those of the rest of the country. The University too was indignant: after all, it did most of the teaching and now here was an outside body being formed with the authority to tell the Senate what to do. As a paper of the day reported, "the medical atmosphere was in a highly electric condition". The situation in Edinburgh was particularly charged, as the most articulate members of the Royal Colleges, such as Simpson, Syme, and Christison, were on the University staff as well, often signing petitions against themselves.

Without getting much assistance from the doctors, thus underlining the fact that steps must be taken at once to organise their profession, Palmerston set up a committee to 'examine the subject of Medical Reform, with a view to a Bill being passed". An eminent surgeon at St Georges Hospital was chosen to preside over the committee. Benjamin Brodie was a man of noted charm and tact, as well as being active politically. He had an enormous practice in London, which yielded him £10,000 a year, mostly in one guinea fees! Brodie had intrigued Simpson with his theories on mind over matter, and Simpson later said that he considered the success of the Medical Act entirely due to Brodie's use of psychology in handling the members of the committee.

Eventually, after years of wrangling, the Bill was drawn up, limiting the right to practise medicine in Great Britain only to people whose names were enrolled on the medical register and giving rulings on what the students should be taught, and how.

Simpson himself had very definite ideas on Medical education. He believed that real learning came from personal experience, that teachers were more important than libraries, and that a living mind had more influence on a student than a dead book. He was worried that students had so much to learn nowadays that the professors would forget to point out to them that there was a patient attached to the end of the sore leg! Mutual respect must be maintained between doctor and patient and this he drummed into his students at an early age. Education, said Simpson, was to teach a student *how* to think, not *what*, and he must be forced to use his deductive powers rather than his memory.

Simpson was determined to bring his weight on the members of the Medical Act Committee and he followed every step of the drawing-up of the Bill. The Edinburgh Royal College of Physicians supported the final Bill, but the Royal College of Surgeons was adamant: its members felt infinitely superior to the doctor with his bag of drugs, and were determined that they would never come under one umbrella. The surgeons were influential, and their spokesman on the Committee and in the House was Headlam. At the eleventh hour he produced a series of clauses that threatened to abort the Bill altogether. Supporters in London hastily sent Simpson a telegram, on receiving which he announced, "I will start this evening for London and try what can be done". On arriving in the capital, Simpson rushed around, seeing his powerful friends, urging them to back the Edinburgh Royal College of Physicians against the Surgeons. Luckily, Walpole also disagreed with Headlam's objections, and the Bill went through the House by a majority of eighty-seven.

As soon as the Medical Act became law, in July 1858, the General Medical Council was established under Brodie's guidance. It represented all the leading medical and surgical colleges as well as the medical faculties of the universities. As Syme had suggested, a medical register was compiled and the removal of a name from it marked the end of a medical career. The Council lost no time in reporting on the teaching of mid-wifery to undergraduate students, and in stressing the value of a written and practical exam, and members of the Council visited the various colleges while the examinations were carried out to make sure that the standards laid down by them were maintained. The Council also undertook the publication of a "National Pharmacopoeia" and appointed Christison to see it through; Christison complained to Simpson that one of his difficulties was that two of the delegates on his Committee could not understand each other, one so broad Irish, and the other so highly English. Christison referred to his undertaking as the Treat of Union between the three countries.

Only now was it really evident why there had been so much opposition to the Bill: many doctors holding important positions in the South had no qualifications whatsoever!

Simpson, as usual, was doing several things at once. Spencer Wells had now returned from the war, and his journal was printing Simpson's course of midwifery lectures in full. The ournal was also publishing a chain of letters concerning the question of the position in which the Royal College of Physicians now stood in relation to the new act.

The editor became somewhat disgruntled with the subject. "I feel," wrote Wells to Simpson, "that the Edinburgh College will vulgarise the Title of Physician, by conferring it upon all our lowest pill and draught mongers (as they are now doing) if every low Apothocary is to be a physician. . . . The feelihg is here that the Edinburgh College is determined to make money at any cost of professional dignity. However, on this and all points I always act upon the principle of equal practice and fair play to both sides and Wood and Gardiner, your opponents, have as open a pitch in the *Medical Times* as Christison or yourself." Referring to Simpson's contribution to the paper, Wells continued, "In passing to a much more grateful subject . . . I have never published any lectures with so much pleasure. You must let me have that for the first number early, as for the larger number printed we go to press earlier than usual.

I did another ovariotomy three weeks ago . . . the patient is convalescent. I do another tomorrow . . . so far my success has been four out of five. But I suppose we can hardly expect it to continue in that proportion."

The word "ovariotomy" is said to have been coined by Simpson in 1845. The classical treatment of a cyst of the ovary was by frequent tappings. Simpson quoted to his students the caes of a Lady Paget, who had 67 tappings in five years, yielding 240 gallons of fluid! There were the heroics of Euphraim McDowell and his patient Mrs Crawford, along with some others in America and several early surgeons in Britain, but, it was Lizars of Edinburgh and Charles Clay of Manchester who refined the operation. Ovariotomy, however, really belongs to Simpson's heyday of the late 1850s and early '60s. He himself performed the operation very seldom. In fact, he had little to do with the formidable gynaecological operations coming into vogue, but he was closely involved with the surgeons who did carry them out, notably Spencer Wells and his own pupils, Lawson Tait, Matthews Duncan, and Thomas Keith. All these men later declared that they were strongly influenced by Simpson's teaching and line of thought in the field of ovariotomy. Simpson's results were far better than Spencer Wells's,

H

whose mortality rate was usually 50 per cent. Thomas Keith
was later acclaimed as the most successful of the ovariotomists,
and his good results attributed both to his technique of cauter-
ising the stem of the ovary and to the fact that his work was done
in a private house in Great Stuart Street, and not in a dirty
hospital ward.

Simpson's own contribution to the surgery of his day was
"acupressure". His nephew Aleck was the first to hear of it. The
new graduate received a letter while studying in Germany.

At present, and for some time past, I have been busy studying
and experimenting upon metallic ligatures as substitutes for
silk and thread in stitching wounds and tying arteries. They
do not irritate and ulcerate like organic ligatures and I do
believe that their introduction will in a great degree revolu-
tionise the treatment of wounds. I fancy I am the first who
has ever applied them as ligatures to vessels laid open by the
course of the knife in the human subject. As ligatures they
excite only adhesive inflammation, not ulcerative, suppurative, and gangrenous inflammation as organic ligatures do. I
find iron and silver wire the simplest, platinum excellent.
Now, I want you to get a view of a work of Purmannus on
Surgery. He practiced in Breslau about 1700 and wrote
various books . . . [he] united wounds of the tongue with silver
sutures. Again, Dieffenbach refers to Sosset using gold threads
in stitching vesico vaginal fistula. Who is Sosset and where are
his papers? Do find them. . . .

"Enclosed are two bits of iron wire used in my experiment." He
had evolved a method of skewering the artery with the metal
wire rather than tying it around. He claimed that this invention
would prevent the type of situation faced by Lord Nelson, who
suffered months of agony as a result of a gunshot wound in his
elbow at Santa Cruz. A ligature tying an artery had included a
nerve, and every day the end of it was pulled in hope of
separating the two, causing Nelson excruciating pain from July
until November. Simpson's suggestion was to replace the use of
ligatures by the technique known as acupressure. In this procedure the needles transfixed and compressed the artery as, to
use Simpson's words, "the stem of a flower is fixed to the lapel

of a coat". Not only was the metal of the needle inert—such as gold or platinum—but it could be easily removed, when the haemorrhage danger was passed, by pulling the end which protruded from the wound. In addition the needle's relatively gentle pressure on the artery did not cause necrosis or decay of the stump retained by the patient. It seemed to Simpson that he had found the answer to the problem of surgical infection. However, aware that the surgeons would take some convincing, especially as the idea had come from an obstetrician, sure enough, Syme, was contemptuous. He publicly declared Simpson's new procedure as "uncalled for, inexpedient, and in most cases impractical".

Simpson coped with the critics of his invention in his usual forthright manner and soon produced a pamphlet, "Answers to the Objections to Acupressure". The Medical Act had forced Syme to accept physicians as colleagues and that was bad enough, but obstetricians, he once said, should be classified with the vets! Syme's dignity was toppled by the thought that Simpson should tell him, a surgeon, what to do and he was furious that "acupressure" was gaining ground in Scotland and France. Also, a few doctors in Dublin were very enthusiastic, praising Simpson in the medical press. Syme was so angered that one morning he startled his students by marching into the crowded lecture-theatre, with a scarlet face and bristling with temper. Under his arm he clutched Simpson's pamphlet. He took a stance in the front of his operating table and, spluttering with fury, denounced the practice of acupressure as "a piece of vulgar insolence", then with one dramatic gesture, he tore the pamphlet in half! He handed the pieces of paper to his assistant, and gestured towards the sandbox, waiting to receive surgical debris and amputated legs. Without another word Syme continued with his lecture.

For the next few days Simpson's lecture-theatre was thronged with students waiting to see the next move. They knew that Simpson would never take this insult lying down. In due course the janitor appeared, bearing a tray, on it was Syme's textbook of surgery. Simpson followed. The excitement among the students was tremendous. On this occasion however, Simpson retained his dignity and without a word, took up his position at his large desk in front of the crowded arena. With a disarming smile he opened the book at a marked page and read the words, "Torn vessels never bleed; torsion does no harm". He then gently closed the book and continued with the lecture.

Simpson publicly pretended to be unmoved by Syme's fury, although he took the opportunity of pointing out in print that Syme's action was hardly ethical or suitable for one of the 24 members of the Council of Medical Education set up to represent the whole country.

Simpson told his own students that he would "be quite content if acupressure begins to be thought of a quarter of a century hence". The influential Spencer Wells, among others, however, championed "Simpson's skewers"; the medical journalist wrote and spoke in favour of acupressure on many occasions.

Modern surgical opinion is that Simpson's idea was a good one based on sound pathological principles. Indeed the technique did enjoy a short vogue. However, with the introduction of absorbable ligatures and aseptic procedures, it soon fell into disguise and Simpson's skewers" were forgotten.

The British Medical Association held its twenty-sixth Annual Meeting in Edinburgh in the last week of July 1858, when it drank to "Prosperity to the approaching birth of the Medical Council of the British Nation". Simpson read a paper on the techinique of acupressure which was very well received and numerous doctors got up and reported on several cases in which they had successfully used the technique.

Simpson wrote to a friend that "the summer of '58 was the brightest and happiest in all my past life". His family was growing up and Queen Street was full of the chatterings of children. Sometimes Simpson would please them all by suddenly darting out of his study, ignoring the waiting patients, shouting, "Come on then, let's go off to Bathgate".

Simpson's nephew, Robert Simpson, Dr Aleck's brother, remembered that

The visits of our famous Uncle to Bathgate were always red-letter days in our lives. He gave my father short notice of his impending visits, and he suddenly appeared in his carriage with its pair of spanking greys and the handsome coachman, George Wilson with a spotted dog in a trap. My father and mother busied themselves with the preparation of a meal to

Uncle's taste, and father gave hints to some of the poor folks who, he knew, would value Uncle's advice; and the "Professor", as he was called, had often a busy time with patients. He catechised us about our work at school and asked us to spell Mediterranean and such a spelling puzzle as "he was engaged in the unparalleled work of gauging the symmetry of a peeled pear". We all made a point of not being far off when Uncle left, because invariably, as he shook hands with us, he had a pleasant way of leaving a sovereign in our loof. This, by Mother's orders, we had to put into our "penny pig" and to spend under her benign supervision.

The Bathgate cousins got on well with the Queen Street children, and visits were reciprocated. Simpson's daughter Eve confessed later that she and her brothers felt far closer to their father when they were little, as then he always had time for a joke and a game with the youngest child. As they grew into their teens, they tended to withdraw from him, all except Jessie. She was the only one of the children who would dare to hide in their father's study and then pounce out as he sat at his desk, or creep up from behind and throw her arms over his eyes, asking him to guess who it was. He was never short with her and always liked Jessie to pour his tea, as she knew exactly how much sugar and which cup he liked. The older children felt closest to their father when away from him: then he wrote down what he had no time to say.

The third-son, Jamie, was born with a skin disease, which was getting progressively worse each year. It was now beginning to creep over his face and he was seldom seen by visitors. However, he was a great favourite with anyone who knew the family well. Simpson searched for a cure for the boy's affliction and his mind was often on Jamie when he read of the treatment of facial sores among the Greeks and Romans. Jamie was a happy boy and liked to make things with his hands, but his father now realised that he was losing his sight. Simpson sent him to London to consult a Dr Startin, under the care of his aunt, Wilhelmina Grindlay. She brought him back three months later and settled in at Viewbank to take special charge of him.

Simpson's compassion stretched farther than his own circle of relations and friends, and involved him in a variety of schemes

for improving the lot of the working class. Many a respectable
guest was taken to see for himself just how dreadful were the
conditions in the Old Town. He subjected the Member of
Parliament, Mr Cowper, to a "midnight ramble" down the
High Street, in and out of the wynds between the tenement
lands towering on either side.

Simpson agreed with William Anderson, who wrote an article
in the *Courant*:

> Much less is known, we venture to say, of the closes of Edin-
> burgh than the interior of Africa; The internal arrangements
> of the Red Indians' Wigwam are much more familiar to the
> Christian public than is the condition of the hovels in which
> many of our townspeople live.

Simpson took Mr Cowper into a narrow close, where they
encountered a woman who showed them "two shirts for the
making of which she would receive 4 pence each, 'For' she
remarked, 'If I ask as much as I should get, people grumble so'."
She was compelled to work the greater part of the night and
lived in a cellar partitioned off with old newspapers over a
wooden frame. She had three children and was a widow, her
husband having died three weeks previously, after years of ill
health and uselessness.

In this tenement a "house (or "flat" as it would be called in
England) consisted of one room. In some of these there was not
space enough for an ordinary-sized man to stand up with his
hat on. The walls were soaked with damp, because there was
never enough ventilation and very often no light at all. All these
rooms "borrowed light", by having windows into the next
room, and the intervening partition stopped short of the ceiling.
Cowper reported that "in two or three instances we found
families of 4–5 living in attics of 4' × 10' and height from 3'–6',
rents a shilling and two shillings a week, paid in advance". The
rents were shamefully high and the poor in these localities were
paying relatively more for their homes than any other class in
the community. The proprietors of many of these tenements
cleared 90–100 per cent profits per year. If the money for rent
was not forthcoming, the tenant had to go and his place was
immediately taken up by another destitute family. Simpson

was among a group of benevolent citizens who attempted to buy some of these properties of 1850, with the idea of forming a cooperative movement, but such an exhorbitant sum qas asked that the idea fell through and the hovels continued to exist, and landlords to profiteer.

There was always a demand for even a tiny space; the effect of the Highland clearances was still sending thousands out of the glens south into the cities, and the potato famine in Ireland was still responsible for labourers sailing for the Clyde and into Glasgow from where they overflowed eastwards.

"Ye ken, we puir folk are ay glad to get in our heids ony-where," said a young girl to Cowper and Simpson, as she clut-ched a baby in her shawl and a toddler by the hand. She lived with eight of a family in one room, taken up mostly by the bed shelf. There was a recess in the back of this room, in which the two visitors from Queen Street found a family of twelve huddled together on some very damp straw. There was no water for either family, and of course, no lavatory. The garbage was tossed out of the door into the passage, where it joined the filth of ages and spilled down the stairs.

One of the worst tenements in the Old Town was Crombies Land, in the West Port. One entered it through a narrow dirty passage that led into a small confined, filthy court, surrounded on all sides by broken down dwellings. This property was not old—in fact, it had been built within the last twenty years, although it looked at least a hundred. A rickety outside stair led up to the first and second floor. There was no light in the court, and there were no windows. In a corner at the back of the open space were two hovels.

In one miserable den lived a widow and her two boys of 8 and 10 [reported Cowper of Crombies Land in the West Port]. No bed, a few dirty rags, showed the place of repose. From the structure of the apartment we came to the conclu-sion that it was a byre. Not being sufficient light for accom-modation of cattle, it had been let for a dwelling house! Floor causewayed and an open drain runs through. To see how much light there really was, a candle was put out and the room then was in total darkness! Light from outside not penetrating farther than passage. Woman paid 9 pence for this and light. She made 2 shillings a week cinder gathering. Children did not even know alphabet.

Simpson warned Cowper that there was still worse to see, and took him to Cants Close in the Cowgate. This, at three and a half feet broad, was the narrowest in the city. The houses on either side were seven stories high. Looking upwards the walls did not seem to be more than a yard apart. The overhanging wooden fronts filled up the narrow space so completely that it was almost impossible for air and light to penetrate.

A woman lived on the top flat who also made shirts. She was paid 4½ pence for each striped garment which, after deducting thread and light, left her 2 pence for eight hours work; so, for a bare subsistence, she had to work eighteen hours a day.

As another letter to the Courant pointed out, "If the Christian community of the town were aware of the appalling conditions in which thousands of children are growing up they would bestir themselves. There is evidently no want of money, a one congregation in the town it appears is ready to give £400,000 for a new place of worship!"

According to the landlords the reason for the poor lighting in the wynds of the Old Town was that Russian sailors came up from Leith and drank the vegetable oil in the lamps! Municipal lighting did not come in until 1888.

Anyone attempting to improve the lot of the poor came up against the whisky. There were 965 shops in Edinburgh where a dram could be obtained for one penny and only one where a cup of coffee could be bought for the same sum. This one shop was in the Grassmarket, and the four shops adjoining it sold spirits. The consumption of whisky was incredible: Simpson put it at 9,623 gallons a year, or 2½ gallons per man, woman and week-old child.

"Whisky shops cause drunkenness, much more than drunkenness demands whisky shops," declared an editorial in the Lancet based on Simpson's information. The fact was that the sale of spirits was the only livelihood of the shopkeepers. There was no profit on sugar, so every little grocer's shop had cheap provisions in one window, and whisky displayed in the other. The Lancet disclosed that most articles sold to the poor were adulterated. Coffee was mixed with acorns. mustard consisted almost entirely of flour coloured with turmeric, and cocoa of flour coloured with earth. Checking up, Simpson bought a pound of "Finest West Indian Arrowroot" at two shillings per pound and discovered that it actually consisted almost entirely of potato flour at twopence per pound.

The Irish labourers in the Edinburgh shows were labelled "a very rough type" and described by one Free Church Minister as being "a pestilence as well as a pest. . . . This country desires and deserves to be protected from them." Simpson remarked that it was a peculiar thing that the Irish did not lose their fertility under urban conditions, and also pointed out how odd it was that a poor starving mother would produce a strapping, healthy child, and could usually provide it with enough milk.

Simpson was also involved with the poor in his home town of Bathgate. The handloom weavers there were out of work: 179 looms were idle in December and, as little work was coming in, 134 others would soon be in the same boat. As the average weekly wage for the past year had been only 5/9d. for 18 hours' daily toil, few families had much "put by". These were actually the last days of the hand looms, the big companies on the West Coast being able to produce woven cloth at a much cheaper rate. But a future for the area was dawning. Simpson was one of several men who realised that there was shale oil, and coal and jobs to be had, in the low, rolling West Lothian hills. A mining company was launched to exploit this natural resource and to give work to the unemployed weavers. To start with, Simpson's "Midcalder Mineral Oil Company" was unlucky and hit poor shale, but it was not entirely a philanthropic venture: during its third year, Simpson's 101 shares yielded him £525 4s. od., and by 1865 the company struck good quality shale from which oil could be refined. But it was an expensive way of procuring oil and eventually the company ran into debt.

Intellectual Edinburgh was buzzing in 1859. Principal Lee of the University suddenly died and, to the consternation of most of the faculty, the scientist Sir David Brewster was appointed his successor. Lord Cockburn had said of him, "You will find Sir David a most pleasing gentleman the first year, a nonentity the second, and in the third a very hell upon Earth." St Andrews University had been in a turmoil during Brewster's tenure as Principal there, but Simpson admired the outspoken scientist. He considered his book on Sir Isaac Newton "brilliant", and was very impressed with Brewster's work on optics, which had resulted in his invention of the kaleidoscope. Simpson, therefore, was delighted with his appointment and offered to smooth their path in Edinburgh. Accepting Simpson's invitation Sir David and Lady Brewster moved into Viewbank until they found a house for themselves in town.

The Principal of the University had no great authority. He received £1,000 a year in return for which he was the spokesman of the professors forming the Senate. In this position he was always listened to and so able to bring great distinction to the University by public speeches, and could also bring influence to bear on the students as they were often in the position of a captured audience.

Brewster was seventy-eight when appointed. "He will sharpen our wits," prophesized Simpson. "Now we might all get some work done."

CHAPTER XI

The Veteran

THE FIRST SPRING of the 60s saw Simpson in Manchester lecturing on Roman colonisation, and a few months later came the publication of his first book on archaeology. In his address to the Society of Antiquaries of Scotland on 28 January 1861, Simpson explained his enthusiasm for his hobby: "Archaeology is the study of man—his ways and works, his habits and thoughts. Down through the centuries, man has scattered behind him his tools and ornaments, his weapons and his religion. The evidence of his march of progress is lying about us. The fascination lies in finding the pieces of jigsaw and fitting them into place." In this address, Simpson gave a rapid sketch of the discoveries of modern archaeologists with such diversions as "Dr Livingston told me that on more than one occasion, when Africans were discoursing with him on the riches of his own country and chiefs at home, he was asked the searching question, "but how many cows has the Queen of England?" Simpson rounded off the address by urging the Society to fight for the preservation of relics, ruins and records of the older days. "The Glasgow–Edinburgh railway had been built straight across the Roman Wall at Castlecary, and the iron road to Carlisle had passed right through the very centre of the ancient stone circle at Shap. A few feet on either side would have preserved this monument. Once the stones were down, no amount of enthusiasm or money could replace them. Vandalism should be a criminal offence. Who are we of this generation to have the effrontery to demolish the heritage of centuries?" Simpson must be turning in his grave now.

At a subsequent meeting of the Society, Simpson read a paper on "The Inscribed Stones of Scotland" that aroused great interest and was, according to Douglas Laing, a very important work. The paper referred particularly to the cat stane or battle stone of Kirk Liston. It was situated near the south bank of the

River Almond about three miles up from the old Roman camp at Cramond. This was the place where Mary Queen of Scots was caught and carried off by Bothwell in April 1576. The stone or monolith, was four and a half feet high and twelve feet round, and inscribed with four lines of Roman letters. Previous opinion held that the inscription commemorated either the Scottish King Constantine IV or a Pictish King Geth. Simpson, however dismissed these theories and produced evidence that it was actually a stone commemorating Vetta, grandfather of the two Teutonic brothers, Hengist and Horsa, who, according to Bede, invaded Britain in the fifth century. Vetta was a Saxon leader who fought with the Picts and Scots against the Romans. The stone is important in that it is a connecting link between the two great invasions of Britain by the Romans and Saxons and marks the end of the Roman dominion over Britain and the first dawn and commencement "of that Saxon interference and sway in the affairs of Britain which was destined to give to England, a race of new Kings and new inhabitants, new laws and a new language".

In his address Simpson urged the Society to make plaster casts of various stones threatened with destruction. In a few instances his advice was taken and the results can be seen today in various museums scattered across Scotland.

Letters came to 52 Queen Street by every post recording finds, or asking Simpson for an interpretation of curious markings on stones. Douglas Laing sent Simpson an old medical manuscript printed in the sixteenth century. He had found it in a bundle of waste paper. A prescription that particularly intrigued Simpson read, "To sartane man sleip till he be Schorne".

In November 1861, much to his delight, Simpson was elected Professor of Antiquaries. His letter to his good friend the photographer Octavius Hill expressed his delight.

Edinburgh 23 November: 1861.

My dear Sir,

Allow me to return through you to the Royal Academy, my most cordial thanks for the honour which the Academicians have bestowed upon me, in electing me their Professor of Antiquities.

In accepting with sincere pleasure that high honour from the hands of a body of my fellow citizens, so greatly and so justly esteemed as members of the Royal Academy, I have only one regret to express, namely, that I fear and feel that my slender Archaeological studies do not entitle me to the office.

But, believe me, you could have elected no one who had more sincerely and zealously at heart the advancement of the love of Scottish Antiquarian Knowledge.

The office has one preeminent attraction, for it connects me officially with The Royal Scottish Academy, an Institution of which any real Scotsman has so many reasons to be proud.

I have the honour to be

Very faithfully yours,
J. Y. Simpson.

Despite his archaeological studies, Simpson was not neglecting his medical practice. His most illustrious patient in 1860 was the Empress Eugénie who came to Edinburgh to consult him, having been told it was impossible to summon Simpson to France. She left Napoleon behind and travelled to Britain by herself. She stayed at the Douglas Hotel in St Andrew Square. For her benefit Colonel Ewart marched the 78th Regiment of Rosshire Buffs, recently returned from India, past her window, with the band playing "Parlant pour la Syrie". The Empress was delighted and leant out of the window, bowing and waving her handkerchief to the soldiers.

The following June Simpson had another important visitor from abroad, the American doctor, Marion Simms. Simpson wanted to meet the American as he claimed to have invented an operation which cured the awful complaint of vesico-vaginal fistula. Simms, whose family came from the back-woods, is said to have had a handsome face, magnetic personality, and a professional manner which a British contemporary described as "very nearly perfect". Although in Scotland he was disliked intensely and was considered vain, women travelled thousands of miles in America to be treated by him.

Simpson was very interested in Simms's background. He was born to a South Carolina farmer, who left his sugar-cane crop, his baby son, and his slaves, to fight the British in 1813. His, mother died from over-bleeding, blistering and purging which may have helped Marion decide to become a doctor. Qualified in Philadelphia, he returned to South Carolina. He had no patients until the other doctor in the community went on holiday. Then two babies fell ill. Both died. Simms was so upset, that he threw his doctor's shingle or brass plate down the well and fled the town. The land of promise in these days was Alabama, so Simms headed there, covering the 500-mile journey on foot. His first patient here died of puerperal fever, and his second protested from his sickbed, "My God, do you call that thing a doctor? Take him away. I'm too sick a man to be fooled with." Success began to come to the young doctor when the settlers joined battle against the Creek Indians. The Creeks were being ousted from their lands by the whites and were now putting up a last-ditch fight. Simms patched up arrow-wounded settlers and bullet-shattered Indians until there were no more Creeks left to fight. However, when the settlers returned to their homesteads and hung their guns on the wall, they began to fall ill. They complained of chills, fevers, delirium, and death usually followed. It was malaria. Most doctors bled their patients. Simms dosed them with the magic drug, quinine, instead, and his clients got better. Simms also differed from other Alabama doctors in that he enjoyed reading the European medical journals and used to ride into the local town of Mont-gomery to get hold of them. In these journals he read of Liston and his surgical procedures for correcting cross eyes, club feet, and hare lips. No one else in the Southern states would dream of treating these, but Simms took these patients on, and quite soon he had a thriving practice. He moved into Montgomery in order to cope with it. Simms was lucky in that he had plenty of material on which to practise and perfect his cosmetic surgery techniques—the Negro slaves.

In 1845 he was aked to go to a plantation a mile or so out of town, where a seventeen-year-old negro girl, Anarcha, had been in labour for three days without giving birth to the child. Simms delivered the baby with forceps and returned home thinking that he had seen the end of Anarcha. But five days later, he heard that the young mother had completely lost control of her bladder as a result of damage from the forceps and the pressure of the infant's head during the long labour. Simms reluctantly trekked back to the plantation and was horrified to see the result of his previous visit. Great holes were in both walls of the girl's vagina, and the damaged tissue was sloughing away. This condition is called vesico vaginal fistula, and is now coupled to the name of Marion Simms. Simms told Anarcha's owner that she was incurable. She could never work for him again nor could he sell her in that condition. She was a millstone around his neck.

It so happened that in three months Simms saw three other negro girls suffering from the same complaint. He refused to treat them. Then a white woman was thrown from her horse when it stumbled over a wild pig lurking in a ditch. The fall left her writhing in agony and Simms was sent for. He had to do something here. A long-forgotten remark by a teacher at his medical college was recalled, and he placed the woman on her hands and knees, which was the classical method of curing a displaced uterus. Quickly her pains ceased. The patient's position created a suction in the pelvis. air rushed in, and Simms suddenly appreciated that he had a clear view into the cavity. As he wrote in his autobiography, "Then said I to myself . . . why can I not take the incurable case of vesico-vaginal fistula, which seems to be so incomprehensible, and put the girl in this position and see exactly what are the relations of the surrounding tissues? Fired with this idea, I forgot that I had twenty patients waiting to see me all over the hills." He jumped into his buggy and drove hurriedly home, stopping at the store of Hall Mores and Roberts to buy a pewter spoon.

One of the negro girls, Lucy, was still in a shed at the bottom of Simms's yard. He hustled her up to the house, put her on her hands and knees and "saw the fistula as plain as the nose on a man's face. . . . I said at once, why cannot these things be cured? It seems to me that there is nothing to do but pare the edges of the fistula and bring it together nicely. . . Fired with enthusiasm by this wonderful discovery, it raised me into a plane of thought that unfitted me almost for the duties of the day."

Needless to say, it was not as easy as that. Simpson, Spencer Wells and many others in Europe were attempting to cure the fistula in a dozen different ways. The German, C. W. Wutzer of Bonn, confessed that during 1838–1852, "twenty cases of the fistula were subjected to 48 operations—among which were leytroplasty, episiorrhaphy, cauterization, sutures, interrupted or twisted or both—and only two cured." However Marion Simms differed from the European doctors in that he had docile negro slaves on which to experiment. Plantation owners were delighted to hand over to him such unprofitable invalids. Simms states himself that he offered the owner of Anarcha and Betsey and another young girl, the following proposition in writing: "If you will give me Anarcha and Betsey for experiment, I agree to perform no operation on either of them to endanger their lives, and will not charge a cent for keeping them, but you must pay their tax and clothe them. I will keep them entirely at my own expense."

Simms operated first on Lucy, on 10 January 1846, and expected at once a magical cure. He failed, "till each one had suffered numerous operations, but all to no purpose". He admitted that the agony he inflicted on the girls was "so painful that none but a woman could have borne it"—a strange contrast in attitude to the sex to that practised and preached by Simson.

For four years, Lucy, Betsey and Anarcha, lived in the garden hut and Simms tried out one idea after another. Silk sutures, silver, gold and platinum were tested, then silver quills and lead quills, but they all caused suppuration. Then by chance he tried the fine brass wire used, according to Simms, as springs in suspenders. On the thirteenth try, the sutures held, and the operation was successful. Anarcha was the first to be cured. This was her fortieth operation. Simms only records his own feelings: he was "elated". His paper on the subject appeared in the *American Journal of Medical Sciences* in 1852. All the essentials for a cure were known, however. What Simms did was to shuffle them into the appropriate combination. He was thirty-two when he rationalised the problem, and produced the cure.

The slaves, having served their purpose, were returned to their owners, Simms sold his practice in Montgomery to his assistant Bozeman, and moved to New York where there were more white patients with money. Here, he opened a hospital entirely for women. Generous support came from the ladies of New York Society and soon the centre had to be enlarged, although Simms said "the medical men of the city called me a quack and a humbug and the hospital [was] pronounced a fraud". The land bought for the overflow happened to contain the mass graves from the cholera epidemic in New York of 1832, and it took all summer to remove the coffins buried in tiers, eighteen deep. 27,000 corpses had to be disposed of.

In June of 1861 Marion Simms decided he needed a holiday and came to Europe. Later he wrote:

In coming to Europe, the man that I most wanted to see was Professor Simpson, of Edinburgh. His labours and contributions to the literature of the day were the most valuable that had been made to the growing science of gynaecology. So, in leaving Dublin, I went by way of Belfast to Edinburgh, where I was warmly welcomed by Simpson, Syme, Christison, and Matthews Duncan. I had performed many of Simpson's operations; I was the first to operate according to his method for dysmenorrhoea. He had represented the operation as being attended with no danger. I had had serious haemorrhages follow it . . . and I thought that possibly I did not perform the operation precisely as he did. So I was anxious to see as much of his practice as I could.

No warm friendship, however, sprang up between Simms and Simpson. Perhaps because Simms instantly became Syme's protégé, but also because Simpson operated on the celebrated fistula by the "Bozeman" technique, using Bozeman's instruments and Bozeman's methods of after-care. Simms claimed that his assistant had stolen his methods and called them his own. However, the fact was that Bozeman had arrived in Europe first, and has impresssed the medical old world with his surgical skill, and successful demonstrations, and was also liked as a man.

Simpson wanted Simms to demonstrate his fistula operation, but no patient could be found in Edinburgh. So Simpson and Christison took Simms for a walk instead. Simms reported that, "Christison was then no longer a young man, but of wonderful endurance physically. I shall never forget his walking me to the top of Arthur's Seat and down again. I was awfully fatigued, but he did not seem to mind it in the least". Simpson remarked that Americans did not seem to have the use of their legs like the Scots, and also took life far too seriously.

Simms was delighted to find that Simpson was not the god in his own country that he was abroad. He wrote in his biography, when discussing the doctors in Aberdeen that:

When I told of my accidents following his operation on the cervix uteri, and that he had none of the sort, they laughed at my credulity. They gave me the name of a doctor living not ten miles distant from the city, whose wife had been operated on by Dr Simpson and she died within forty-eight hours afterward. Of course, this surprised me exceedingly, and when I returned to Edinburgh, I spoke to one of the eminent surgeons of the town, who was a friend of Dr Simpson's and not an enemy—for the doctors of that city seemed to be divided into two classes, those who were the friends of Dr Simpson, and those who were not—and this gentleman told me that he knew of one death following the operation, and that in Dr Simpson's own hands.

Simms passed this gossip on to friends in Dublin who said on hearing it, "We did not tell you before you went to Edinburgh, for we saw that you had an exalted opinion of Dr Simpson and his work, and that to such an extent that we were not disposed to spoil your ideal of the man."

Proceeding to London, Simms demonstrated his operation to, among others, Spencer Wells. Simms recorded that, "my operation was a great success, but the patient died". He hastily left for Paris, where he again performed his operation, and was invited to carry out his procedure on a young countess. Her first child had been born when she was nineteen, two years previously, but was a stillbirth. The baby's head had been malformed and its birth had resulted in the dreaded fistula. She was under the care of the renowned French surgeon Nelaton who corresponded frequently with Simpson, and who had operated on Napoleon and Garibaldi. It was he who suggested that the Empress Eugenie travel to Edinburgh to consult Simpson. Simms recorded that the countess was,

. . . young, beautiful, rich, accomplished; and, as Dr Nelaton
had told her six months before that she was absolutely incurable, she was praying for death, but in vain, for patients
seldom die of afflictions of this kind. In all my experience, I
have never seen a case of this kind which was attended with
such extreme suffering. She was obliged to take anodynes in
large quantiies to relieve the pain attendant upon sufferings.
She passed sleepless nights and restless days, and was
altogether one of the most unhappy women I have ever seen.

As Simpson had noticed, Simms was far from modest, and he
readily claimed now that he could perform a perfect cure. He
asked a Dr Campbell, a socially accepted accoucheur in Paris to
assist, and Dr Nelaton looked on. Simms only allowed his private
patients chloroform, which Campbell now administered to the
young countess. The operation began at 10.00 a.m. Simms
reported that,

Forty minutes later, I asked Campbell if the pulse and
respiration were all right; he said "Yes, all right; carry on".
Scarcely were these words uttered when he suddenly cried
out, "Stop, stop! No pulse, no breathing." And sure enough
the patient looked as if she were dead. Dr Nelaton was not in
the least disconcerted. He quietly ordered the head to be
lowered and the body to be inverted, that is, the head to hang
down while the heels were raised in the air.
    . . . My notes of the case, written a few hours afterward,
make it twenty minutes that the patient was held in this
position. . . . The time was so long that I thought it useless to
make any further efforts, and I said "Dr Nelaton, our
patient is dead, and you might as well stop all efforts." But
Dr Nelaton never lost hope, and by his quiet, cool, brave
manner he seemed to infuse his spirit into his assistants. At
last there was a feeble inspiration, and after a long time
another, and by and by another; and then the breathing
became regular. When the pulse and respiration were well
re-established Dr Nelaton ordered the patient to be laid on
the table. This was done very gently, but the moment the
body was placed horizontally the pulse and breathing
instantly ceased. Quick as thought the body was again

inverted, the head downward and the same manœuvres as before were put into execution.

After many minutes of this, the countess breathed again, but the moment she was placed flat, the same thing happened, and the drama was repeated for the third time. Simms said that she looked the picture of death, but at last they heard,

> . . . a spasmodic gasp, and after a long time another, and after another long interval there was a third, and then a fourth more profoundly; there was then a long yawn, and the respiration after this became tolerably regular. She was held in a vertical position until she in a manner became semi-conscious, opened her eyes, looked wildly around, and asked what was the matter. She was then and not until then, laid on the table, and we all thanked Dr Nelaton for having saved the life of this lovely woman. In a few moments the operation was finished but of course without any more chloroform.

Simms was able to write the next day that, "she is now bright and cheerful, hopeful and happy, thankful and joyous". The countess has gone down in history as the first patient to recover from an overdose of chloroform. Dr Nelaton had made his discovery that inverting the head was an antidote for chloroform poisoning, because he lived in a house on the Quai Voltaire which was infested with mice. Great numbers were caught in traps, and then the doctor was in the habit of covering the trap with a napkin and pouring on chloroform, as an easy death for the mice. He found that if then carried to the dustbin by the tail, they would miraculously revive!

Simms had never been an enthusiast for chloroform, and was even less so now. He called the drug "delicious and dangerous" and wrote to America, "I am done with chloroform, and will never again operate on any patient under its influence, and believe it ought to be banished from use." Simms returned home but America was in a turmoil, and he rushed back to Paris to avoid the Civil War. There he set up a thriving social practice, and charged $1,000 for his vesico-vaginal cure. One of his patients was the Duchess of Hamilton, who gave Simms a château to live in at Baden Baden for the summer while he treated her complaint. During that summer the Duke of Hamilton fell downstairs, and after three days died. His constant nurse during this time was the Empress Eugénie. She liked Simms and became his patient, although she later said that "he had not the gentleness of Simpson, nor the humour".

After his American visitor had left, Simpson dashed over to Ireland to attend the Social Sciences Congress. In an interval between lectures he sauntered in the Phoenix Park with William Wilde who was accompanied by a lady friend. Suddenly, round a graded walk, came Simms. Simpson was amused when Wilde greeted the American with, "Why my dear fellow, is that you, you great unshaven humbug?" Wilde then invited him to dinner, but Simms refused, pleading lack of time to change. "But," said Wilde, "it is you that I want and as for your coat you may pull it off and hang it on the back of your chair and you may turn your breeches wrong side out, if you will, but I must insist on you wearing them."

Before the year was out, Prince Albert was dead. Sir James Clark was blamed for not realising that the prince had typhoid. Simpson, who had been fond of Prince Albert, nevertheless wrote Clark a letter saying he at least appreciated his difficulty as the prince always thought he was ill, and was the classic hypochondriac.

Simpson was particularly low at this period and the death of Albert seemed to upset him more than one might expect. He wrote some sad poems which he had printed privately. The fly leaf bore this explanation: "Isle of Wight, writen during some unnaturally Spring like weather at end of 1861 when the country was in its first darkness of its National Loss, and the New Year threatened to open with the most sanguinary of modern wars (U.S.A.)." The fifth poem expressed his feelings on the American War.

> Since it is War, my England, and nor I
> On you nor you on me have drawn down one
> Drop of this bloody guilt, God's Will be done,
> Here upon earth in woe, in bliss on high!
> Peace is but mortal and to live must die,
> And, like that other creature of the sun,
> Must die in fire. Therefore my English, on!

And burn it young again with victory!
For me, in all your joys I have been first
And in this woe my place I still shall keep,
I am the earliest widow that must weep,
My children the first orphans. The divine
Event of all God knows; but come the worst
It cannot leave your homes more dark than mine.

Various philanthropic works interested Simpson at this time. He helped draw up plans for a cottage hospital at Newhaven, and suggested a vegetable shop where the locals could bring their own produce to sell and so learn to grow greens. Cabbage and peas were unheard of among the poor and even kale was eaten more by cows than by people. Simpson also remarked that a few flowers growing around in the cottages would gladden the heart and do even more good than a fresh green. Simpson was constantly approached to put his name to similar schemes, and was even persuaded with difficulty to lay the foundation stone of the Free Church at Armadale, a mining village near Bathgage. He was late and arrived in a cloud of dust after a large crowd had collected on a fresh breezy afternoon between squalls of rain. A minister present wrote of the scene.

None who listened to the impressive tones of that soft silvery voice can ever forget the occasion. The marks of mining enterprise were all around him, under his eye hundreds of upturned, earnest faces of hard working men; many tears on cheeks unwont to weep, and his native Bathgate Limestone Hills lying in rounded beauty in the distance—as he talked of the hard but noble struggle which falls to the lot of working men.

Simpson was now fifty. At this point in his life he began to question the meaning of the Bible. Dr Guthrie, the Free Church leader, had inspired him with the "Fire and Brimstone" type of Old Testament religion, but Simpson was unable to tie this up with the work of the Scottish geologist, Lyell, or Darwin's *Origin of Species* which he had been constantly in his mind since its publication in 1859. His archaeological research left him well informed on the other religions and he once remarked that, "if all the church men say is true, how did the Chinese get so far in their civilisation without Christinaity?" He was fumbling for an explanation of life when he realised that young Jamie, his third son, was going to die. Jamie was fifteen, and during the last few months had become an ardent believer in the simple Christian faith of the Sunday School Mission variety. "I am going to Jesus," were the child's last words to his father who knelt beside his bed holding his hand. Simpson, heart-broken and ill with a throat infection wrote to a friend of Jamie's last days,

> He had a most kind French "bonne" taking care of him and trying to teach him to speak French; and my assistant Dr Berryman and he were great companions. He taught him latterly turning and carpentering, for though half blind, he worked away wonderfully and greatly by touch, making boxes, desks, cages, etc. . . . for his little brothers and sisters. He had the garret room over my bedroom fitted up as a workshop and as I was laid up latterly with this sore throat, the knock of his busy little hammer and the burr of his turning lathe were somehow pleasant sounds. They are all silent and still there now, and I listen to them in vain.
>
> He died most calmly and peacefully on Sunday morning, and just as he breathed his last breath, the church bells began to ring.

Simpson's search for an intellectual explanation of Christianity seemed to cease with Jamie's death, and he now accepted the simple teaching that his boy had believed in. On the tombstone that he had placed over the tiny body of Maggie in 1844 was inscribed, "Nevertheless I live", and as Simpson wrote in another letter two days after Jamie's death, "it seems to me, that we have somehow a greater interest in Christ's Kingdom seeing that my dear Jamie is already there".

In February 1862 Simpson gave his first religious lecture. The subject was "God is Love", and it was delivered to an audience in Bathgate. In March he repeated it to a packed meeting in the Queen Street Hall. An old woman in the audience was asked what had struck her most in the evening. "It was before the meeting began", she answered. "It was the smile on the face of the gentleman in the chair."

On the 20th of the month he addressed a gathering of enthusiastic medical missionary students. "I am the oldest sinner and the youngest believer in this room." he announced, and went on to testify that he had joined the ranks of the converted and from now on would trust in Christ without asking why.

The Carruthers Close Mission, numbering well over 2,000, met on a Sunday night in the Free Church Assembly Hall. For the next few years Simpson frequently presided over the meeting. His conversion caused much comment, and several of the audience attended specifically to see "how Simpson looked as a Christian". The report was made known, however, that he was Simpson still. Simpson did nothing by halves, and he expected others to be as enthusiastic. He had no time for "easy ozyness" as he put it. "We had a minister yesterday", he reported, "but oh cauld, cauld, why will not men speak as if they believed what they said and wished others to believe it? Just look at Guthrie—what zeal, what fire". This simple, cheerful faith did not last for long. By 1866 Simpson had become involved in an obscure doctrinal argument with a leading theologian, the Rev. Sir Henry Wellwood Moncrieff. Simpson had been invited to become a church elder, which involved signing a declaration of acceptance of the Westminster Confession of Faith. Simpson felt unable to do this, and he expressed his reluctance to Moncrieff. His chief objection was that the Faith stated that the world existed only six days before the appearance of Adam, some 6,000 years ago, and Simpson considered this absolute rubbish. "I do believe," he remarked, "that the works and the word of God will never (when they are both fully understood) contradict each other. The Bible, however, as it always seems to me teaches us no kind of knowledge which the intellect of man is unable to discover. It is a revelation of religious truths, not a revelation of scientific truth; and when the Westminster divines insisted their opinion of the duration and age of the world, they took up a position in science which science has since entirely contradicted."

Simpson accused the clergy of apathy. They continued to teach the old doctrines that modern studies of evolution now proved quite untrue. However, despite these reservations,

Simpson remained a practising Christian for the rest of his life.

Simpson's nephew, Aleck, was now one of Simpson's three assistants in his practice. His own son David, a tall, handsome, but serious boy was a medical student and he spent every spare minute with his father. Simpson sent him to France in the summer of 1863 to polish up the language and gain medical experience. He joined his son for a few days in July.

David, writing to his sister Jessie, complained that he had great trouble keeping up with their father who left five minutes for a meal between breakneck visits to hospitals, museums, and drawing roms, and that he felt quite ill with the noise of people talking to his father. While the rest of the party argued about what they would do next, Simpson was up and ready and half way there. David was apparently quite taken aback by the esteem in which his father was held abroad. He told his sister that people even offered to press his clothes. He refused, although, as David remarks, his coat needed it badly. On a visit to Paris Simpson was received in Madame Victor Hugo's salon. "The excitement was something tremendous", related David, "and for a time you could hear the sound ss-ss-ss-running through the room as there passed from mouth to mouth the exclamation, 'C'est Simpson, C'est Simpson!'"

Another doctor from a little village near Aberdeen, recorded that a letter of introduction from Simpson was an open sesame to the greatest possible kindness and attention in Paris.

The sparingly emotional Velpeau brightened up when he was informed of the source of my credentials. Paul Dubois was equally demonstrative. "And how is Dr Simpson?" he inquired in his slow measured English, "Is he very busy?" "One of the busiest men in the world, I will venture to say," was my reply. "It is his nature to be busy," rejoined Dubois— "He could not exist if he were not busy."

At this time in Edinburgh there was among the enthusiastic students who clustered around Simpson to watch him operate one who stood out particularly—his name was Lawson Tait. Tait was a flamboyant, blustering, dogmatic young man, who grew up to take an important place in the growth of gynae-cology. He liked to be different and, presumably in order to

draw attention to himself, he claimed to be Simpson's illegiti-
mate son. There is no record of Simpson denying this, but
equally there is no record that this claim was ever made before
Simpson's death. Tait's very able biographer, I. Harvey Flack,
M.D., states categorically that Tait's father was an Edinburgh
lawyer and that he was born on 1 May 1845 at 45 Frederick
Street. There is no record of Tait's birth in Edinburgh, but it
was not compulsory to register births in Scotland until 1855, and
before that many families connected with the disruption of the
church would not have their child baptized in the Church of
Scotland. These births were therefore not recorded in the local
registers that were subsequently taken over by the Registry
Office when it came into being.

A student of Tait's in Birmingham towards the end of the
century wrote that Tait made a point of often mentioning "That
great man J. Y. Simpson," at which the students knowing the
rumour of his illegitimacy would clap and stamp. Tait enjoyed
this, and would pause and bow his head, then cast a knowing
look around the hall. . . .

At the time of Tait's birth, Simpson's adored first child, his
darling Maggie, had died. He was striving to cope with his
growing practice and teaching commitments; he was short of
money; his wife was pregnant again; and he published three
very heavily documented papers in five months. It can surely
be accepted as highly improbable that he had either time or
inclination to become embroiled in a love affair with an Edinburgh lawyer's wife.

However, Tait admired Simpson enormously, and Simpson
approved of the alert young student, and fostered his enthusiasm
by suggesting lines of research and giving him anatomical
specimens on which to carry out experiments. Simpson was
working on acupressure at this time, and Tait carried out
practical tests with acupressure methods on twenty-eight arteries
of healthy cats and dogs, verifying his results by comparing
them with human vessels given him by Simpson. Tait published
his results in the *Medical Times* in 1865. Tait qualified in 1866,
and left Edinburgh to become a great surgeon. He was square
and hairy, and when a close friend, T. P. O'Connor, commented in 1885 that he looked remarkable like Simpson's
statue, then erected in Princes Street, Tait "volunteered to

make the statement to me that the story true and that he came of perfectly respectable, though not distinguished parents".

While Simpson was giving time to this precocious young student, he was also concerning himself with the course of the American Civil War. Slavery was absolutely wrong, he insisted, and Lincoln must be supported. In '63 and '64 he corresponded in detail with friends and patients in the Northern and Southern States and paid the paper boy a half guinea in order that he came first to 52 Queen Street when on his morning round. Simpson was fascinated by America. He mentioned in a letter to a J. H. Conklin of Houston, Texas who had borrowed £2,000 from him when stranded in Europe, that it was remarkable how speedily America had swallowed up the civilisation and cultures of ages past and spat out a clean and new virile form of man. What a future! He said he himself was too sentimental to move to the States, but he urged his son David to go.

Towards the end of 1864 Britain was hit by an outbreak of cattle plague, or foot and mouth disease. The disease swept over the Lammermuirs and into Scotland. The farmers were small in the North; Simpson's father, for instance, had owned three cows, but many people had only one. If this beast died, there was no milk or meat for the family, for there was seldom any money to buy another.

Simpson had recently become interested in a method of preserving meat. Three-quarters of the weight of water was driven off at a low temperature leaving the outer constituents unchanged; "concentrated meat extract", he called the final product, which he considered to be of particular importance just now when hundreds of thousands of cattle were dying of the plague, and the shortage of meat was becoming acute. The situation was getting desperate in Lowland Scotland. Simpson received numerous letters from farming friends and local doctors beseeching him to do something about it. His mind turned to vaccination, and he immediately wrote to the Cattle Plague Commission in Victoria Street, Westminster, for some facts. The reply stated that the Commission had dismissed vaccination as too expensive, but mentioned that Russia had recently established some "Inoculation Institutes". Simpson at once dispatched a battery of letters to the British Ambassador in Moscow, to the Principal of the Moscow University, and to

Russian doctors in twenty-five different hospitals; he also got in touch with numerous travellers who might have contacts in Russia. He sifted the answers and made his conclusions known to the Commission in London who replied that they still considered that inoculation was not successful enough to warrant the expense. On receiving this negative reply. Simpson made his amassed facts known to the public via the press, who then agitated for the Government to take steps at once to make inoculation available to the farmers in spite of the opinion of the Cattle Plague Commission.

Simpson's evidence showed that inoculation of oxen from the Steppes significantly reduced the mortality rate, but that it was not successful with other breeds of cattle until the third generation. The London Commission was not encouraging, so Simpson formed an Edinburgh Cattle Plague Committee, with the purpose of trying to find a disinfectant that would destroy the virus. The Committee also aimed to inform the farmers of available treatment and advise them on how to prevent the spread of the disease, for Simpson saw no future in a body in London with no lines of communication with a farmer in, for instance, an Argyll Glen.

In the spring of 1865 Simpson sent his second son, Walter or Wattie, as he liked to call him, abroad. In a letter to Wattie he wrote,

> The longer I have lived, the more I have regretted the state of my knowledge of spoken French, German, etc.; and in all professions the knowledge of languages every day becomes more and more indispensable, because the new discoveries, and disquisitions on them, must be read in various languages to enable those running in the race to keep up the required pace.

Wattie went on walking tour through the Pyrenees to Spain and then over to Alexandria. From there he wrote home asking for £20 in order to buy a horse. Unfortunately, he bought a bad one, and it sprained its ankle on a stony path. Wattie spent three weeks in a remote village, living off dates, waiting for the horse to recover. On hearing this, Simpson sent him £25 with instructions to spend it on learning about horses before he invested in another beast. Wattie replied "I shall try and buy a 'Carvases' (Policemen's) horse. They are the best to buy here. You may be sure I shall be very careful for £20–25 one gets a nice horse and a hardy one. Most of the Carvases having native Egyptian Steeds." Wattie added in a postscript. "I have got your cigarette machine for which many thanks. It is very ingenious, would be useful for any one who had not fingers. It was a great puzzle to find out how to use it. We had good fun trying."

When Wattie returned to Edinburgh, a ball was arranged to welcome him home. On the day of the dance, at the end of a lecture to a crowded hall of students, Simpson suddenly invited the entire class. The students were delighted and clapped and cheered and all agreed to come. Returning home to lunch, Simpson casually mentioned that he had doubled the number of guests. Jarvis, the butler, was flabbergasted, and Miss Grind-lay, who was managing the household affairs, became scarlet in the face and speechless. Simpson could see no difficulty. Eve, remembering the occasion, said that her father merely told Jarvis to clear out another flat, get more musicians and double the order for food supplies, remarking firmly that he would "welcome every one of my class, and see they get dancing and supper galore".

David graduated as a doctor at the end of the university session, and Simpson now sent him across the North Sea to glean experience in the medical centres of Europe. David wrote to his father from Prague. "We arrived here on Tuesday night, expecting every few miles we journeyed to be stopped by snow, but fortunately no such calamity befell us. It was bitterly cold, however, as you can well imagine. Prague is really a lovely place. . . . We walked out to the Jewish synagogue which they say is the oldest in Europe. It is a curious very small building. The walls have not been cleaned for 400 years with the exception of the lower 6 or 7 feet which are under water when the river overflows."

David went on to describe and draw an obstetrical instrument used to remove a baby, dead in utero. It differed from the one that Simpson had evolved and David told his father it was more efficient and simpler to use.

A month later David wrote from Berlin. He was now working

in the Charite which had forty beds set apart for diseases of women.

The chief Doctor [wrote David] has been uncommonly kind (a rare quality in a German) . . . Perhaps the arrangements in regard to the beds might interest you. The mattresses are composed of cloth sacks stuffed with clean straw; the bed cover being a double fold of blanket in a linen bag, like a pillow case. The women are not delivered in the same bed they are to lie in. After every delivery, and whenever a patient is discharged, the mattress is destroyed, i.e. the straw is thrown away, and the sack washed and refilled. In consequence of these precautions Dr Martin has only had five cases of puerperal fever, during the time he has had to do with the hospital. No cyanide of potassium, or other chemical agent is used in cleaning the hands; only soap and water.

All women who wish to be delivered in the institution must give notice at as early a period of their pregnancy as possible, and they are promised a bed on condition that they come to be examined about once a month between that time and their full period. By this arrangement a capital opportunity is afforded to study the size and situation of the uterus and the state of the vagina and cervix during the various stages of pregnancy.

He always used china specula and Kiwisch's uterine sound. This week he's been going largely into anteversion; without differentiating between it and autoflexion. He gives four causes for it; first in virgina; excessive growth of the back wall of the uterus, 2nd the placenta being situated on the back wall and imperfect involution of the site of its attachment taking place. 3rd inflammatiory contraction of the round ligaments (Virchow) and 4th inflammatory contraction of the sacro-uterine ligaments; the last being the most important.

Cephalaematomata he looks upon as reaching a crisis and commencing to retrograde about the 9th or 10th day after birth and invariably opens them on the 11th or 12th day by lancet puncture. Some times but rarely the cavity refills with serum which he evacuates in the same way. He has never had a case go wrong and suppurate.

In the Charite he showed me a very interesting case of

cancer, which had entirely destroyed the perineum and recto-vaginal septum.

I took tea with his family on Friday night and was very kindly received.

Langenbeck had an excision of the wrist joint this week, the first he has performed since he came to Berlin. The operation was very skillfully done.

David came home in March, and joined his father in the practice. He was soon a great favourite with the patients, who were as happy to see him as they were Simpson himself. David set to work to organise his father, and for the first time appointment books were seen in Queen Street. Simpson had always claimed that the chaos of snippets of paper and random notes or loose pages strewn around his study were actually quite rational and that he could put his hands on what he wanted at once.

In August of 1865 Simpson became ill. He complained of pain in his side again, and frequent headaches. After three weeks in bed, he went to the Isle of Man to stay with Captain Petrie. David was left in charge at Queen Street, and he also attended to Simpson's commitments in the Lying-in Hospital. Jessie took the opportunity of bringing in the painters, which made it, as David complained to his father "uncommonly uncomfortable" in the house.

Simpson was well and back again in Edinburgh in time for a busy winter. The New Year opened well for him. An embossed ivory envelope arrived at Queen Street from Lord John Russell who wrote on behalf of the Queen. The Crown was offering Simpson a baronetcy, in recognition of his professional merits, especially the introduction of chloroform. On reading the letter Simpson at once sat down to write to his brother Sandy. "I do not know whether you ought to condone with me or congratulate me. But most unexpectedly this morning I received from the Queen the offer of a Baronetcy, Lord John accompanying the offer with very complimentary observations. I fear that I must accept. But it appears to me *so* absurd to take a title. I have not spoken of it here yet. Do not mention it."

On two previous occasions Simpson had been offered a knighthood, but he had refused to accept. He was not the first to decline a knighthood: William Cheselden, the London surgeon who died in 1752, refused one from Queen Caroline on several occasions and Dr John Hall, Shakespeare's son-in-law, also refused to kneel to the sword, preferring to pay James I £10 for turning down the offer. But a baronetcy was something different, and Simpson was the first medical man practising in Scotland to be so honoured. He accepted, though reluctantly.

However, as word of the baronetcy became known, letters of congratulations began to shower into Queen Street and visitors queued up at the door. "All Edinburgh has been here," said Jessie with pride.

Wattie was abroad again and Simpson wrote to tell him of the news.

> Edinburgh, 9 January 1866.
>
> My own dear Wattie,
>
> I do not know whether you have heard or not that, as a New Year's gift I had a present sent me, which, since it has become known has set all Edinburgh apparently mad with joy and congratulations. I have shaken hands daily till my arm is weary and sore. The proudest of all about the gift is your uncle in Bathgate. At all events, he is a thousand times prouder of it than I am. In fact, when the gift was first offered me I was rather ashamed to speak of it and doubted about accepting it. But it was decided at last otherwise. But the gift itself was right Royal and came from the Queen herself. It was in short the offer of a Baronetcy and I suppose I ought to esteem it greatly as I am, it seems, the 1st Scottish Professor as well as the 1st doctor in Scotland who ever received that rank from the Crown. The offer was made in such very kind and gracious terms that it was difficult to refuse . . . everybody pokes at me their "Sir" which I would be glad to avoid. It seems to have caused much joy not only in Edinburgh but everywhere around. But my paper and time and subject are done.
>
> Dear, dear Jessie (daughter) becomes weaker and weaker but is as gentle and good as ever—more gentle and wetter.
>
> Believe me, your loving father,
> J. Y. Simpson.

The Queen's gift of the baronetcy pleased the newspapers, and all carried leaders on Simpson. Even the *Lancet* was enthusiastic and commented that Simpson deserved the distinction on several counts, quite apart from his promotion of chloroform. The Lancet concluded by stating that Simpson's reputation was European, and the honour fully deserved. American, French and German medical journals were equally delighted and congrautlated the Queen rather acidly on deciding for once to confer the distinction on someone who was worthy of it.

Simpson now had to think of some armorial bearings. His mother's family, the Jervaises, carried a coat of arms, and Simpson decided to base his own on this. For the crest, he chose the rod of Aesculapius over the motto, *Victo dolore*, and this he would hand down to his oldest son.

Meanwhile, Sir David Brewster, Principal of the University, along with the current presidents of the Royal Colleges, decided to organise a public dinner to show their appreciation of the honour conferred on Simpson. The Earl of Dalhousie was enthusiastic and preparations went ahead.

Then, suddenly the plan was cancelled. Simpson's oldest son, David, was dead! The blow stunned Simpson. He took to his bed, allowed only his old friend Mr Pender in, and ate nothing. It was two days before he could write to Wattie.

16th January 1866.

My own dear Wattie,

I have to write to you grevious, most grevious and heart rendering news . . . God has called dear dear Davie home to himself. . . . It is needless to say how utterly overwhelmed and crushed we all feel, and I have got out of bed chiefly to write you these dreadful and melancholy news.

I never knew how very very very dear he was to my heart till now he is gone from us for ever. . . . My darling little Jessie is greatly broken down with this catastrophy. She is very helpless in bed and would allow no one to dress her sores but Davie. 'Gentle Davie', as she declared no hand to be so soft and kindly as his. I greatly fear you may miss her also when you come home, unless you come very soon.

Mamma, Jessie, Willie, Magnus and Eve all join in overflowing love.

Cordially, your ever affectionate father,

J. Y. Simpson.

I

The promising clever young doctor David died at the age of twenty-four, of appendicitis. A month later Jessie, aged seventeen, followed her brother to the grave. Simpson's sunbeam, his darling daughter with the beautiful long auburn hair, was gone too.

Letters of condolence from all over the world were even more numerous than had been those of congratulations on the recent baronetcy. These letters now tended to come from more ordinary people. They could understand death, whereas a baronetcy was part of the life of the aristocratic. One of thousands is from a lodging house in Glasgow, scrawled on a dirty scrap of paper—"I am so sorry for you, Mary Ellen".

The Victorians at least had the satisfaction of mourning, and people were allowed to grieve, and talk out their sorrow. "I felt this Baronetcy such a bauble in health", wrote Simpson, "and now, when sick and heartsore, what a bauble it is."

The tragedy drew what remained of the family closer together, Wattie and Eve desperately trying to fill the gap. Simpson's reaction was to bury himself in work. He was up as early as usual, and read for most of the night. After fourteen hours or so in his practice, he found time in the evening to follow up various projects. He was currently engaged in work on waterproofing material. His shale company could now produce oil, but were not quite sure what to do with it, so during February and March Simpson contacted numerous cloth manufacturers, and sent them samples of the "Midcalder" product, with a view to their using it to make cloth impervious to water. The difficulty with the Bathgate oil was that it failed to dry properly on the material and did not have the body to fill up the pores of the cloth enough to make it waterproof. The reply from the textile factories was, in fact, that linseed oil was more satisfactory and cost less. But Simpson would never accept defeat, and simply cast his net further afield. Eventually an American firm was found that would buy the oil, and Petrie's ship carried it across the Atlantic.

During the summer of 1866 Simpson persuaded the University authorities to install a restaurant where medical students could procure a good wholesome cheap meal, with speedy service. The alternative was a slice of unbuttered bread in an ale house, or nothing till the end of the day when they retired to their lodgings for a finnan haddie.

The year 1866 also saw Simpson interesting himself in the question of education for young boys. He felt that modern languages were more important than the classics, and should have a place in a school curriculum. Science should also be taught, astronomy and biology particularly and each subject by a specialist. As there was no school in Edinburgh with this approach to education, Simpson enthusiastically agreed to put up some of the capital for one to be established.

Simpson was very intrigued by a visitor he received in the early summer, Signorina Jessie White Maria, who had nursed the sick and wounded in Garibaldi's campaign. Simpson called Maria the "Italian Miss Nightingale". Italy and Austria were about to go to war over the possession of Venice, and she had come to Edinburgh to ask advice on setting up a field hospital. Acupressure seemed the answer to emergency amputations, and Simpson also advised her on dressings for surgical wounds. He felt that it was better to apply a thin layer of wet gauze or lint to the surface rather than wads of gutta percha and bandage which kept out the fresh air. Maria complained to Simpson that during the campaign in Sicily more than three-quarters of the soldiers operated on woke up half way through their operations! Simpson put this down to scrimping on the chloroform, and not allowing enough time for the patient to be fully anaesthetised before the surgeon commenced work.

Maria and Simpson also discussed the 1866 folklore of Sicily, where the classical stories were still heard. Simpson became interested in the superstitions and folk cures of Britain, particularly those still practiced in the Shetland Isles. He tried to obtain information via the local ministers, but found that the people were unwilling to communicate on the subject with the representative of the church! So Simpson wrote directly to the fishermen, shepherds and crofters, and sent one of his assistants, a Dr Black up to Yell as an amanuensis. Dr Black reported that sea shells were still considered far more successful at treating a variety of ailments than doctors, and that surprisingly few people came to him for medical attention.

In the early summer Simpson heard that his property in Tobago was losing money. In 1859 Simpson had invested £3,000 along with a Mr O'Neal, who put down an equal amount, and they bought a sugar plantation between them.

Simpson signed a document in 1859, stating, "I leave the direction of this estate entirely in the hands of O'Neal, and guided in all things by his judgement." Unfortunately, the rum produced as a by-product for the estate appeared to contain lead. Simpson suggested new machinery for the sugar-cane squeezing plant, but O'Neal spent the money set aside for this on a boat for himself. Simpson became interested in the question of lead, and cited incidences of it polluting Roman water supplies, and Victorian households. He looked into the production of rum in other Caribbean Islands, and corresponded with property owners in British Guiana and Surinam.

In 1866 the estate lost £3,400 and Simpson decided to sell out. Wattie wanted to go to Tobago and see what he could do, but Simpson refused to let him and sold to the brother of his friend Mr. Pender, at a substantial loss.

In June Simpson received a letter from the Vice-Chancellor of Oxford University, with the information that the degree of D.C.L. had been conferred on him. Simpson went to Oxford to receive the degree, and made full use of his three-day visit by, as he wrote to his daughter, "covering all the colleges of antiquarian interest—that is, all the colleges—boating—listening to the incredibly beautiful boys choir, dining in an atmosphere I would like to see among our own lads here—looking at a Roman fort—and so much besides".

Following this, on the fourth day, Wattie joined his father at Devizes. They swallowed a hasty lunch, then hired a carriage to drive to Avebury to see the stone circle, returning at 11.00 p.m. By 6.00 next morning they were on their way to Stonehenge, then back to Devizes for a standing lunch before catching a train to Bath. Arriving there in the evening, they immediately hired a carriage to drive to some other standing stones some miles from Bath. On getting back to the hotel at 11.00 p.m., Simpson found a telegram calling him to a case in Northumberland. He lay down for an hour or two, then caught the 3.00 a.m. train to London. He took a quick breakfast in London and then continued directly to Northumberland. After seeing his patient he filled in the time before the Edinburgh train by visiting a Roman fort. He eventually reached home, full of enthusiasm at 2.00 a.m. Wattie had meanwhile retired to bed from exhaustion!

Interest in his own University led to another row the following month. The Carruthers Close Mission had established a
dispensary for the poor, staffed by medical students in their free
time. A notice advertising the Mission and its work was hung
on the gatepost of the University. An officious professor, Wilson,
took exception to this and demanded that it be taken down on
the grounds that it did not concern the University. The Mission
turned to Simpson to champion their cause, and he rose to the
occasion. He pointed out to the Senate that as the University
recognised the certificate of the dispensary they could not
refuse the hanging up of the advertisement. The Senate disagreed on principle, and insisted that it be removed at once.
Hearing this, Simpson turned on his heel, summoning a student
with a hammer, and marched down the steps to the janitor's
office at the gate, to nail up a larger notice himself. Christison
remarked that, as the janitor was a friend of Simpson's, that
was the end of that.

In September Simpson was ill again with a constant severe
pain in his leg. The University granted him leave of absence,
and his lectures were delivered by a Dr Keiller. Agonising pain
in his side and severe rheumatism in his legs forced Simpson to
lie on his back in bed. His zest for life seemed to have drained,
and he told his son Wattie that he never expected to rise again.
He could not move without intense pain, and dared not turn
in bed without a whiff of chloroform. This fit of black depression
lasted until October. Then one morning he startled the household by giving orders for two secretaries to be summoned at
once; to these he dictated a manuscript for an archaeological
book on ancient engraved stones, which was published the
following year and dedicated to Sir David Brewster. Simpson
was particularly interested in the cup and ring marking found
on stones scattered throughout Britain, made, he considered,
by a pre-Celtic race—the same people who hunted whales in
the Firth of Forth with harpoons of deer horn in single-tree
dugout canoes.

Simpson was back delivering his university lectures after
Christmas, although his leg gave him such pain that he could
only walk by leaning heavily on a chair that he pushed in front
of him. He found it impossible to climb the stairs to his own
lecture theatre, so he swapped with Professor Christison, who

had his on the ground floor. The students gave Simpson an enthusiastic welcome and told him of a rumour that his absence was due to an enforced stay in Morningside Asylum! Simpson quashed this by producing the manuscript of his book and pointing out the academic labour involved in its conception.

In the Easter holidays of 1867, Simpson decided to go for a "quick invigorating scamper" to Switzerland, stopping off on the way to visit the Paris Exhibition. Mr Pender accompanied him, together with Wattie and a young friend, David Brown.

They spent a happy week in Paris, although Wattie complained in a letter home that his father would be up by 6.00 a.m. and then spend an hour trying to stir the rest of the party. He and Brown had difficulty escaping from the two older men, who spent hours and hours immersed in the antiquarian and art pavilions at the Exhibition and expected the younger boys to be as enthusiastic. When not at the Exhibition they drove about at high speed, sight-seeing. Wattie wrote:

Once or twice my father got me out about 7.00 a.m. to go with him on a prowl as "interpreter". One of these mornings was spent in a surgical instrument makers, where my father gave and received a good deal of information.

On another morning Wattie left the hotel with his father before breakfast to visit one of the hospitals. After going the round of the wards along with the students, they joined the throng in the operating theatre. The surgeon was reducing a dislocated leg on a patient under chloroform. After manipulating it successfully, he turned to the audience and gave a eulogy on the benefits of chloroform, pointing out that in this case the drug also served the therapeutic purpose of relaxing the muscles in the leg. When he had finished, Simpson stepped forward out of the crowd of students, and handed in his card. "Ah Simpson, Mon Dieu, Mon Dieu!" caried the surgeon and flung his arms round the professor's neck, much to the amusement of Wattie and the excitement of the students, who heightened the drama with cries of "Bravo!" and "C'est le hero!"

After this, the surgeon led the visitors to a book shop where he and Simpson became so engrossed looking at old second hand volumes that Wattie thought he would get no tea let alone breakfast or lunch! However, Simpson eventually saw and heard the Wattie's appetite was getting out of hand, and reluctantly agreed to leave.

Once away from Edinburgh, Simpson had made a miraculous recovery, and it was obviously a very happy party that took the train from Paris to Geneva. Wattie wrote home,

A good deal of chaff used to pass between us two juniors and our seniors; they lecturing us about smoking too much and us accusing them of eating too much. At every station we stopped a few minutes. Mr Pender and my father were promptly inside the refreshment room taking coffee, milk, soup, wine, or whatever was going!

We spent a lovely spring day in Geneva strolling beside the lake and visiting various friends of my father. My father that day composed a little hymn which was afterwards set to music. . . .

It was too early in the season to go to Chamounix so we set off early next morning by rail for Neuchatel. There we spent the night. Mr Pender was in the habit of getting the landlord of the inn to bring us a bottle of any particularly fine "wine of the country" he has. My father was very careless as to what he ate and drank and I remember at Neuchatel he shocked us by saying that vin ordinaire and water was much nicer than the "grand vintage" which the landlord produced.

On Tuesday evening we reached Berne, and visited the bears, etc. Our starts were always very early, and my father's occupation in the morning was knocking us up. He was always ready long before the time lest we should be late. I used to tease him by pretending still to be in bed long after I was up. That day, by train and steamer we reached Interlaken. In the afternoon we drove up to Grundenwald very slowly as my father stopped the carriage often to question and examine persons with goitre whom we chanced to meet. Next morning we went by steamer to Giesbach—crossed the lake and posted (9 hours posting) by the Brunig to Lucerne. This long drive was made very pleasant by the endless anecdotes my father told and Mr Pender was so exhilarated that he began to sing snatches of songs, a thing, he said he had not done since he was a boy. Next day (Friday) we went up the Lake of Lucerne staying some time at Altorf.

The party continued to Zurich, where Dr Keller, the leading archaeologist of the city, took them to see some Stone-Age flax thread, cloth and looms, then on to tour the churches. Simpson told Jessie, "I became medical for 10 minutes yesterday and asked Dr Keller to take us to a cutlery shop. They had five sets of obstetrical forceps, and showed me mine, telling us it was 'Sampson's'. Dr Keller was greatly amused at finding I was a doctor as well as a pseudo-archaeologist. He had been reading a paper on chloroform last week, and then it suddenly struck him that my name was connected with it."

Safely home again, Wattie remarked that his father and Mr Pender were refreshed and vigorous after the holiday, but that he and Brown were utterly exhausted!

In the summer of 1867 the question of Scottish representation in the English House of Commons came up once more. The Lord Provost called a public meeting, in the Queen Street Hall and the crowds of interested citizens were so thick that the overflow had to stand in the street and listen to the speakers through the open windows. Simpson rose to talk on the subject of University representation in Parliament, but was so frequently interrupted with applause that the newspaper reporters found it difficult to hear whether his speech was for or against the extra member of Parliament!

Babies were born at home in the nineteenth century, unless one was poor and destitute. An obstetrician therefore spent a prodigous amount of time in other people's houses. The ladies would urge the doctor to come in plenty of time, but inevitably Simpson, for one, always had other things to do up to the last minute. When called to the country he would rush down from his consulting room, leaving a crowd of patients, swallow a cup of tea (or leave it if hot) tear open the bag of instruments put ready for him, find, always, that something was missing, and send the cluster of servants, assistants and family hurrying to search for it. Simpson would stand at the door, his long sealskin coat over his shoulders, clapping his hands slowly and loudly. "Come now," he would bellow, "Come along, I can't wait." Some patient, usually a frail young matron, would run down the stairs and interrupt begging him to listen to just one word. Simpson was adamant, "I *cannot* stop my dear," he would say with a charming smile, and then rush off out of the door held by the butler and heave himself into the carriage that the coachman already had on the move.

Although Simpson dealt with an enormous number of patients, he tended now to hand on those needing an operation to his colleagues or assistants. A patient from England consulted him on the 7 March 1867, and, on deciding that she had a large tumour on the ovary he asked his ex-assistant Dr Keith, to perform the operation to remove it, explaining that "he did not feel strong enough yet for additional work, and the anxiety of the surgical operation'.' Simpson had accused Keith three years previously of "unprofessional conduct" over the case of a Mrs Edmonston who had died as a result of an operation that Simpson felt should never have been performed and had had nothing to do with the aspiring young doctor since that occasion. However, Keith had now proved himself an extremely able ovariotomist, and Simpson was prepared to overlook the previous argument for his patient's sake. Keith felt differently, and he sent Simpson a note from his house at 2 North Charlotte Street, refusing to see the patient, owing to the grudge he bore for "the way in which you have spoken of me for a long time past". Simpson was indignant. He immediately reiterated the case of Mrs Edmonston and justified his accusations at that time. This was that Keith had proceeded to operate on Mrs Edmonston against Simpson's advice and had not informed Simpson of his intention, nor had he told Simpson of Mrs Edmonston's dangerous condition preceding the operating, and did not summon him until she had died.

Keith on the other hand, felt that this was quite unfair, and that he had operated to the best of his ability, and that, having done so, the patient was his, and there was no cause for him to inform Simpson at all.

Both parties now bolstered up their statements by producing witnesses and collecting evidence. Soon half the medical profession in Edinburgh was involved and legal advice was sought. Christison tried to soothe both Simpson and Keith while Syme fanned the sparks.

Some of Simpson's energy during the months the controversy raged was diverted to a patent that he had filed in February 1867. The aim of the invention was to use a jet of oil to produce heat and light. The lamp ran on shale or coal oil which was sucked out of a reservoir and forced through a series of minute holes which were surrounded by a tube of atmospheric air, driven by a suitable fan. The force of the air was intended to break the jet of oil into minute particles so enabling it to ignite and burn. Simpson felt that this method of lighting would be eminently suitable for the Old Town, and at the problem of the thirsty Russian sailors would be solved. The idea was taken up by an Edinburgh firm, but came to nothing.

In August the Medical Association met in Dublin. Simpson attended, and also received the honorary fellowship of King's and Queen's College of Physicians of Ireland. Syme and Spencer Wells were also presented with the same distinction. The Irish President took it upon himself to attempt to bring Simpson and Syme together, but Syme would have none of it, and Simpson was indifferent.

Simpson was made much of in Ireland, as he wrote to Jessie. "In Dublin every person was kinder than another. In all meetings I had the seat of honour thrust upon me which involved a good deal of speaking. But I was in the spirit of it, and when the struggle came. . . . Between English, Irish and Scotch speaking, Scotland (so they averred) was not last. We had a great dinner of nearly 300 doctors. I was placed at the side of the President (Dr Stokes) and had to drink his health."

Simpson escaped from Dublin for three days' stay at Dromore Castle, Kerry. He and his host made an excursion to the Bishop of Limerick, taking their own salmon and lamb which they cooked in the Bishop's kitchen. Simpson recounted the day:

The Bishop . . . carried me off to the mountain moors and showed me there some stones and rocks marked with the cups and circles that I have described in my work. . . . It was truly "eerie and awesome" to see them in that distant locality, ancient sculptures so very like those I had seen in Northumberland and Scotland, that truly they looked as if they had all been cut by the same hand. To discover some of them the Bishop had removed 4' of turf accumulated on the bare face of the sculptured rocks.

It was dark when Simpson and his party left to return to Dromore Castle, so the Bishop lit a candle and balanced it on the top of his episcopal hat to light the way to the beach. "As we rowed off," wrote Simpson, "the shore party sang a most beautiful and wild parting song, to which our boat party duly replied."

Simpson returned home for three weeks' hard work but was back in Ireland in September to deliver a long address to the Social Science Association in Belfast. In his paper Simpson declared that Lying-in-Hospitals should be completely scrapped and rebuilt as complexes formed of little independent pavilions, thus preventing the spread of epidemics. This idea startled the audience and caused much comment in the press. Meanwhile, his family were spending their holidays in the Isle of Man.

Simpson was disappointed that no letter awaited him on his return to Queen Street so he sat down to write himself to his daughter.

3rd September 1867.
My dearest Eve,

Of course there is no ink in that barbaric Isle of Man or you would have written since long ere this time. Try pencil. It will do quite well . . .

What is Willie doing? Has Magnus committed many murders with his gun or rod? What is the "firstly of woman kind" herself doing in the Old Isle of Man?" [Simpson went on to describe the latest dog addition to the Queen Street household who was turning out to be a very devoted assistant in the practice.] His last occupational rights consist in carrying up to bed some thin book or other for him and me to study. Up stairs he marches most proudly with it in his mouth,—bending his back and wagging his tail at such a furious and frantic rate that I sometimes fear for him, book and all, all rolling backwards. He visits all the patients, but instead of feeling their pulses and asking them to put out their tongues, he smells at them and sometimes touches and licks their ear. Then when he and I get back into the carriage, his first occupation generally consists of butting up and trying to take my nose into his mouth. When kept at home from rain or other causes he howls piteously and is always behind the door barking vociferously when I return. He attends all the consultations regularly every afternoon. Sometimes he sits in my chair looking wise and every inch a doctor. Sometimes he jumps into the patient's chair and hangs his head seemingly unhappy and distressed. Latterly he has got a chair of his own and which Barbara (the maid) has spread with a luxurious rug. There he lies, hour after hour watching all that goes on from the corner of his eye.

At this moment I am writing at the desk in the dining room window and he is lying at my feet, rolled up between the two front legs of the desk. Today I was very tired and did not rise till 11, which he did not object to. I saw a little sickly child who screamed (out at Newington) whenever I spoke to it. But I took the dog up on my knee and then he and the child played together till I got its pulse and he all examined. That is one of the uses of the dog—assistant.

But my paper is done and I must stop. Wattie is to be with you on Tuesday.

Your ever affectionate father,
J. Y. Simpson.

Only a few weeks after this, in September 1867 Lister published his revolutionary paper in the *Lancet* on the use of carbolic acid to destroy the lowest forms of life.

In the *Lancet* of 2 November, Simpson reviewed Lister's communication in his own paper "Note on the History of Carbolic Acid and its compounds in Surgery prior to 1867". Simpson's mind was still fully occupied with his own brainchild acupressure, and he felt that if only surgeons would adopt the use of his pins, there would be no need for Lister's carbolic acid.

The winter passed in lectures on archaeology, acupressure, suppuration and cancer cures and one on education, in which Simpson pointed out that neither Dickens, Bunyan nor Shakespeare had studied the classics, and yet all wrote tolerable English. He disapproved of the theory that Latin and Greek trained the mind, and felt on the contrary that they stunted and deformed it. Memory was all that a study of the classics cultivated, and left quite untouched the higher powers of observation which were far more necessary for a scientific future.

In December Simpson's investments in the shale oil project collapsed, and between that and his Tobago property, he lost a great deal of money. He wrote a sad letter to Wattie, now at Cambridge, apologising for squandering money that he should have put aside for his heir. Wattie remarked that it was quite out of character for his father to value wealth, and reminded him that he had often said that he did not want to handicap his children by leaving them too much.

Simpson was back in form for a meeting of the Edinburgh Royal Society of 20 January 1868. At the December meeting he had been chastised for his use of the word "pyramid" in connection with a tomb in Ireland, by Professor Charles Piazzi Smyth. Smyth was the professor of Practical Astronomy at Edinburgh, the son of a naval captain who surveyed the Mediterranean. He was interested in the pyramids, particularly the great pyramid of Cheops. This was by no means the largest or most impressive of the monuments, but had been singled out for attention by a long succession of inquirers, including Herodotus, Isaac Newton and more recently a London publisher, John Taylor. Taylor believed that Noah had supervised its building, and that the rather bizarre proportions were due to the use of the biblical measure, the "cubit". Smyth took up this idea and wrote five books on the subject. He insisted that by a complicated mathematical formula, he had identified the cubit of ancient times and he went on to explain that twenty million of these cubits laid end to end would equal the length of the earth's axis, and that the distance from the earth to the sun was exactly one thousand million times the height of the pyramid. Smyth next showed how a tourist with a measuring tape could pin down the dates of the Flood and even the Creation. He asserted that British weights and measures, derived from the cubit and the pyramid-builders' inch, were divinely inspired. The scientific world was not quite so enthusiastic, and Simpson, devoted his address to the Society in January to demolishing Smyth's pretensions. After cataloguing arithmetical error and other irregularities Simpson declared with mock solemnity that the brim of his hat was equal to one twenty-millionth part of the earth's polar axis. As Professor Smyth himself described the scene. "The pretended measurement was performed on the hat, in place of the sacred cubit of Moses as determined by Sir Isaac Newton; and performed with so much unction of manner and look as to be received with cheers by the large and learned audience."

In early February Simpson's friend Sir David Brewster, Principal of Edinburgh University, died at the age of eighty-seven. In April Simpson wrote to an old assistant "The public, not myself, have set me forward as a candidate for the Principal-ship; but I have not yet applied. Professors Christison, Syme, Playfair, etc., all started. But I believe it lies at present between me and Sir A. Grant of Bombay, who will not take it unless he gets the vacant Moral Philosophy Chair also. The time of election is not fixed and I will not be greatly disappointed if it does not fall on me."

At first Simpson remained on the sidelines, but with his eagle eye on every step as the plot unwound.

The Professors of the University wanted Christison to be Principal, and their spokesman, Professor Lyon Playfair, reported to Christison that Simpson had come to him and said "It is all nonsense the idea of my being made Principal. It is supremely ridiculous, Dr Christison should be the man."

However, Simpson was a favourite with members of the Town Council, who always liked to point out that they had elected him to the midwifery chair against the wishes of the University. The Council had a say in this election too, and they disliked Christison, who fought their domination over the University. The Town Council and his other friends decided to secure the appointment for Simpson, however, and as the excitement of partisan feeling grew, Simpson found that he wanted the position for himself after all.

The other candidate, Alexander Grant was little known in Edinburgh, so Simpson characteristically set to work to ferret out his past. Grant was said to be the most eminent living writer on ethical science. He had taught moral philosophy at Oxford before becoming Professor of Philosophy and Political Economy at Bombay, and Vice-Chancellor of that university. Wanting some personal details, Simpson sent a telegram to a business man in Bombay, the son of the Rev. Dr Brown of the Free New North Church in Edinburgh. The answering telegram read, "An indifferent churchman. Broad religious views. A popular lecturer. Caution in the use of this." Simpson unscrupulously made the most of this information. He later stated that he and his supporters exploited the statement purely in the interest of religion and Presbyterianism. Simpson reasoned that "Of course Grant should not hold the Moral Philosophy chair if his religion was indifferent, and, if not the chair, he should not be Principal."

Meanwhile, Christison met Sir Alexander and liked him immediately, and felt that he indeed should be the candidate. Christison withdrew his own name, and put all his weight and influence to the support of Grant. Christison wrote to his son "You will be surprised to learn that I have had Sir Alexander Grant for a dinner guest yesterday, and that we may be said to be at once intimate and cordial."

Syme, needless to say, also supported Grant. In fact, so did twelve members of the ■■-strong Senate. Their tactics to undermine Simpson's cause were to murmur about "the sealed documents that Christison had handed over reputed to contain defamatory evidence of a moral nature", and to write anonymous letters to the *Edinburgh Courant* signed "Lynx". Private letters were published, personal remarks made known, and moral and religious characters defamed all round. Simpson's supporters said that Grant was a slovenly and ineffectual speaker, while Christison and Syme warned that Simpson, if elected, would bring in an element of discord fatal to the efficiency of the University. They pointed out that Simpson was not on speaking terms with many of his colleagues. "Oh!" Simpson was quick to reply, "Syme himself does not speak to six of his colleagues in the Faculty of Medicine!"

The good citizens of Edinburgh, however, were so convinced that Simpson would be elected, that the Scotsman took the matter for granted and announced in the paper of 10 June that Sir James Simpson had been appointed Principal.

To save the University from such a calamity, the professors drew up a protest and presented it, with twelve signatures, to the University Court on 18 June. This succeeded in postponing the election, and Simpson's supporters took the advantage of time to draw up a testimony of their own. In three days, they had this signed by nearly one thousand graduates of the University from all parts of Britain. It stated that "It is our earnest and decided opinion that the office of Principal should not be bestowed on an utter stranger, unconnected with the University and totally unacquainted with the workings of the Scotch University System". Simpson however, was a distinguished student and professor of the University who had already done much to uphold and extend its reputation and he "is at this moment, in our opinion, one of the most earnest and indefatigable workers for the intellectual as well as physical improvement of his fellow men. We consider that his election will not only add lustre to the University, but be highly advantageous to the interests and prosperity of an Institution, whose fame and well being we have all deeply at heart."

When the election day came, much was the same as when Simpson aspired to the Midwifery Chair in 1840. The Lord Provost rose to his feet, and proposed Simpson. He endorsed his vote by saying that,

In the first place, Sir James Simpson is a person who has been known to us all our lives. He is an esteemed citizen of Edinburgh. He is a man who has attained a high reputation as a medical and scientific discoverer. He has received distinguished honour from Her Majesty; and he is a person of sufficient fortune, as I understand, to enable him to do those hospitalities that are required of a Principal. . . . Recently there has been an inquiry as to how much work a professor actually carried out as some were believed to have no students whatsoever. Now I think that in putting Sir James Simpson at the head of the senatus we are facilitating inquiries of this kind. He is a person so estimable and so well known for the uprightness of his character, that he will be disposed to see that the affairs of the University are administered correctly and in such a way as will be satisfactory to the University Court as well as to the public generally. There is one reason why I would not put stress on the objections which have been made to him. I could make statements in opposition to remarks that have been made on this subject; but I think we should not go into any of these petty objections; I think it would be much more preferable that I should confine myself to what I have said. I therefore, adhering to my expressed opinion and promise, have much pleasure in proposing that we proceed to this election; and I beg to nominate Sir James Simpson as Principal of this University.

However, the Lord Justice General then rose to propose Grant, and was seconded by Sir William Gileron Craig, who said, "I think that in the appointment of the Principal, who is to conduct the affairs of the University, you must take care that these affairs shall be conducted not only with discretion but with good feeling and harmony among the members of the Senatus. That is a matter which cannot be over-looked." Grant was obviously more acceptable to the Senate, considering that the members included Syme; Smyth, the astronomer; Henderson, the homeopathy exponent; the Professor of Divinity who was horrified at Simpson's questioning of Genesis, and his refusal to sign the Westminster Confession; and the Arts professors all of whom advocated a classical education to the exclusion of anything else. Considering the opposition, it is surprising that Sir Alexander Grant was elected by only a majority of one.

An editorial the following day remarked,
The appointment of Principal to the University will long be remembered in the annals of intrigue. This is what we have got by confiscating the patronage of the University as held by the Town Council—and we all know the Bombay educationist, for this is a man back again from Bombay, the place to which we have long been accustomed to consign our clever second-rate men; and instead of him we might have had one whose fame has spread as far, not as that of this unknown translator of Aristotle, but as far as that of Aristotle himself has. What Sir James Simpson has done for Edinburgh and the University, no one required to be told. In what way Sir Alexander Grant is ever to attract to it a single student, we are utterly unable to conjecture. He represents a condemned system. He is out of the march of the age.

On 1 August, at the close of the University session, it was Simpson's turn again to deliver the graduation address. It was his twenty-eighth year as a professor at Edinburgh University.

The theme of his address was the value of self-education, won for oneself, and its limitless possibilities. "In some professions one has to think—in others, one has to *do*. Medicine calls constantly for both, plus the ability to feel. But don't expect much gratitude from your patients," he warned the new graduates. "Man is a thankless lot."

The excitement of the medical profession lay in new discoveries and research. Soon, predicted Simpson, there will be no measles or smallpox, and tuberculosis would be blotted out. The new ophthalmoscope revealed the secrets of the eye and the laryngoscope the interior of the throat. More was bound to follow in this field "Possibily even, by the concentration of electrical or other lights, we may yet render many parts of the body, if not the whole body, sufficiently diaphanous for the inspection of the practised eye of the physician and surgeon."

"There will be few of us here left in fifty years," warned Simpson. "Life is short. Our hearts have beaten seven thousand strokes since we entered this hall that they will never beat again. We are all seven thousand pulse beats nearer death."

The students loved this and gave Simpson a standing ovation when he sat down.

Meanwhile the Town Council decided to confer the Freedom of the City on "Sir James Young Simpson of Strathaven, Bart., M.D., D.C.L."

At the presentation the Lord Provost pointed out that it was quite unusual for a man of Simpson's reputation to have remained in Edinburgh, and not followed the brain drain south. In his reply Simpson quoted the complaint uttered on the occasion of his succession to the Chair of Midwifery; the business men felt that Simpson would never draw patients from other parts of Scotland as had Dr. Hamilton. "But, I think", said Simpson, matter of factly, "that this prophetical objection has been fully gainsayed, for I believe I have had the good fortune to draw towards our beloved and romantic town more strangers than ever sought it before for mere health's sake." Simpson was right: patients and practioners had come from America and Australia, India and Africa, as well as Europe. But he was dissatisfied: "Sometimes when I look back and reflect I feel regret and dismay that my avocations and my idleness have prevented me from doing more."

The fact that Edinburgh had recognised him, pleased Simpson more than all his foreign honours put together. He knew only too well that the prophet is seldom respected in his own town. However, the Lord Provost's speech stirred up all the old controversy over the rights and wrongs of using chloroform in childbirth, and now also the U.S.A. tried to embroil Simpson in their Wells versus Morton and Jackson arguments that were still going strong, on the question of priority.

Simpson was in good health now and revelling in his baronetcy and the influential and political friends with whom he now mixed. He had stopped attending religious meetings and his old lightheartedness had returned. This was his entry in a young girl's autograph album at this time:

Questions and Answers
1. Put on your wishing cap and what would you wish for?—the recovery of the idle past.
2. Gather your favourite flower—forget me nots.
3. Name your principal tastes—Auld nicknackets' stones and books and (tell it not) a cup of tea.
4. What time of year would you prolong?—New Year
5. Choose a motto—Excelsior.
6. Where is the pleasantest spot in memory?—any spot, neither bells, messages nor telegrams can reach me.
7. What do you think the fittest subject for reform?—Ladies dresses without a doubt.

Simpson's serious interest in reform now again involved him in the battle for the recognition of women doctors. Queen Victoria, had been brought into the world by a woman doctor, Marianne Siebold, as her mother had no confidence in British medicine, but even so, she herself was all for keeping women out of the professions, especially medicine. In 1870 she enlisted Gladstone's aid in squashing the appeal for woman's enrolment in the London hospitals.

Now that Simpson's interest was roused he began to consider the place that woman doctors had held in the past.

The Greek Gods had women doctors. Hygiea and Agamede of the golden hair tended the civil population, and like women ever since, stayed at home to tend the sick. As civilisation advanced, the medical profession developed, and learned men came to the fore, but all around the world there were countless homes where people were born, lived and died with only such help during illness as could be given by the women of their communities.

The University of Salerno saw the light first and had women on its faculty from the birth of its medical school, and from then on in Italy the doors of the University have been open to women on the same terms as men, although for hundreds of years comparatively few were educationally qualified for admission. But this was far from the case in Britain or the New World.

However, as the nineteenth century progressed, the "woman" movement was gaining strength on both sides of the Atlantic. Medical service, which called for a medical education, was an important element in the revolutionary trend. There were women agitating everywhere. Elizabeth Fry in the prisons in England, Lucretia Mott among the slaves in the States. The First Women's Rights Convention was held in 1848 in New York. Two years later in the autumn a medical college entirely for women opened in Philadelphia. In common with many manifestations of early women's liberation it had the support and backing of the Quakers.

Elizabeth Blackwell, as has been seen, was the first woman doctor that Simpson met. She later told him her story: how one morning in October 1847, the Dean of 'Geneva College", Dr Lec, had assembled the entire medical school, and, hands trembling and voice shaking, had read them a letter. It was from a doctor in Philadelphia who wrote that a young girl who had been acting as his apprentice would like to be admitted to their college. She had applied to every other Medical School in the United States and they had all turned her down. Perhaps though, as Geneva was in the country, it might be less prejudiced? There was not a sound in the hall when the Dean had finished reading. The boisterous students were speechless: Dr Lec then announced that the faculty had handed the decision over to them. The students were to cast a vote, and it was to be unanimous. One negative vote was all that was needed to bar her entrance. The Dean then fled.

That evening it was the faculty's turn to be speechless. The students had voted "Yea!"

Elizabeth Blackwell was eleven when her father had uprooted the family from England and taken them to America. He was attracted by the free thought and democratic ideals of the New World. On finding that in some ways America was more prejudiced than England, he was soon in the thick of the abolitionist movement. He believed in educating his daughters as well as his sons, and the Blackwell girls studied maths, Latin and astronomy as well as French and the piano.

Behind Elizabeth's fragile appearance was a cast iron will. When she was seventeen her father suddenly died and within two weeks she had turned the family home into a boarding school, bringing in enough money to support the other nine children as well as her mother. After six years of teaching, by which time the family was on its feet, Elizabeth was well aware of the problems that faced a girl looking for an education. Yet it was these practically unsurmountable difficulties that fascinated her and made her decide to study medicine.

It took Elizabeth three years to collect enough money, and to browbeat a college into accepting her. But on 7 November 1847 she walked into the classroom at Geneva. One of the men later remembered that entrance.

She was quite small of stature, plainly dressed, appeared diffident and retiring, but had a firm and determined expression of face. Her entrance into that bedlam of confusion acted like magic on every student. Each hurriedly sought his seat and the most absolute silence prevailed. The sudden transformation from a band of lawless desperadoes to gentlemen by the mere presence of a lady proved to be permanent in its effect.

Finding patients for her clinical study at the college presented problems for Elizabeth, but eventually she managed to wangle entrance to the grim Blockley Almshouse at Philadelphia. In the summer of 1848 it was packed to its grimy rafters. It was the time of the Irish potato famine and boatloads of migrants had made the ghastly journey across the Atlantic only to succumb to typhus on reach the country of their dreams. Hundreds upon hundreds of victims were brought to the Almshouse, racked with the fever. By the end of the summer, Elizabeth had seen so many cases that she chose typhus as the subject for her graduation thesis. This was so good that it attracted attention, and the National Medical Association felt obliged to lift the censure it had levelled at Geneva College for enrolling a woman in its Medical School. To Elizabeth, however, their degree was not nearly good enough. She determined to come back to Europe and learn some more. Paris was hostile, but London friendly, and she settled there for two years. Among her friends was the young Florence Nightingale, and at Lady Byron's house one evening, she met Simpson. He talked with her of her struggles and told her that he believed that women had a place in medicine. Elizabrh returned to America, where she faced her biggest challenge yet. She was now ready for patients but they were not ready for her; nor could she persuade any of the desperately short-staffed hospitals to give her a job. She took to writing to pay the rent, and her common-sense ideas on education for girls soon attracted the attention of a group of intelligent and influential Quaker women, who became her first patients. With this small private practice behind her she felt that she could ignore the establishment, and she opened her own little clinic in the worst slum area of New York. Here, three days a week and on any night that she was needed, she treated migrant women and children who otherwise could have lived and died without receiving the slightest attention from any medical service in the city. It took six years of combating prejudice before Elizabeth's clinic blossomed into the New York Hospital for Women and Children, supported, again, by the Quakers and by the more flamboyant enthusiasm of two New York papers—the *Times* and the *Tribune*.

Meanwhile Elizabeth's young sister Emily had decided to follow in her shoes. Remembering Simpson's kindness and sympathy, Elizabeth now approached Simpson on her sister's behalf. He replied that he would be delighted to receive the girl in his house an as assistant. Emily enjoyed her stay in Edinburgh, in spite of much good natured teasing from Simpson himself.

Simpson was prepared to encourage women and could see that an adequate medical education must be available to them, but he was one of the few. Christison was adamant in his disapproval of female doctors and by far the majority of university senates in Britain felt the same. The doors in England were firmly closed to them, but a chink was discovered in Scotland at St Andrews where in 1861 a sleepy janitor handed out a class ticket costing £1 to a determined young woman, Elizabeth Garrett. Sophia Jex Blake was the first to try for place at Edinburgh. She knew that Simpson would be an ally and, sure enough, wrote that he would be very glad to see her. Professor Masson also wrote cautioning Sophia that "not all of Edinburgh is as liberal as my friend Sir James . . . I fear that at present the chance of the throwing open of professional education and degrees are not so great with us as (you) seem to imagine." Sophia was undaunted and immediately came North and lodged her official application for admittance to the University class.

Now Christison was a member of every influential committee on the University and he determined systematically to baulk Sophia at every step. Simpson however rallied to her side, and Sophia wrote to her friend Dr Sewall on 21 March 1869:

I was sitting yesterday morning at Sir James Simpson's breakfast table, between him and his wife and he passed the paper to me. He was, of course, quite favourable to my application, and I am to breakfast to him tomorrow and hear what he will do about it. He is going off to Rome for a trip this week but I am very anxious that he should vote in my favour first. He is so unreliable that I do not know how to make sure of his doing it though . . . very likely he will be at the other end of Edinburgh when the meeting is held. I told him that you remembered him and always spoke of his kindness to you. I am not quite sure if he recalled it. He spoke kindly of Dr Emily Blackwell.

The Senate in Edinburgh procrastinated. They hedged by saying that they could hardly go to great trouble to organise classes for just one girl. Sophia immediately mustered a band of five other enthusiasts and returned to the fray. The people and press of Edinburgh were by now intrigued and rather amused by the attack on the venerable gentlemen by a small fierce bevy of girls. Sympathy was definitely on the female side, even *The Times* and the *Lancet* rallying to their cause.

Sophia did win the day and the girls were, for the first time in Britain, officially enrolled as medical students at a university. However, Christison was indignant and made life as difficult as possible. It is a pity that Simpson did not live to hear Christison inciting his students to bar doors and hurl mud and abuse at the girls, for he surely would have intervened.

In the spring of 1869, the year of Sophia's triumph, Simpson went to Rome. His friend Mr Pender accompanied him, along with Simpson's daughter Eve. The Channel boat carried a party of pilgrims and as Simpson wrote, the "air was heavy with the soft rich brogue of the South of Ireland". One priest had not had a holiday for nine years, and was in seventh heaven with delight at his journey." Simpson was as excited with his visit. He rushed round the ruins and museums, paying particular attention to the Roman's plumbing and sanitary arrangements. He went to church and on the way watched the Pope, in gala procession, leave the Vatican for Sopra Minerva Church. It was the Feast of the Annunciation, and the streets were thronged with pilgrims, who combined sight-seeing with religion in an enthusiastic way. Simpson also visited the silent empty Protestant burying ground, on a sunny morning at 7.00 a.m. where he walked about the overgrown paths, and cleared the weeds off Keats' grave. He arranged for this and another (that of Dr John Bell) to be maintained, leaving £300 for the purpose, to ensure that they did not fall into disrepair again.

Simpson had many social engagements in Rome but was particularly thrilled with archaeological jaunts to Romulus' wall round the Palatine Hill.

He returned home tired but immediately involved himself in his practice and a new paper on the question of hospital reform. There was much discussion in Edinburgh at this time on the siting and plan of the new Royal Infirmary and on how it should be built. Simpson had been mulling over the problem of hospital construction for many years. As we have seen, as far back as 1848 he suggested small units to prevent cross infection, and had tried to unravel the reasons behind the fact that patients survived operations in their homes or in the cottage hospital far more than in a city infirmary, in spite of the better diagnostic skill and operative dexterity to be had in the latter. Statistics that he had gathered proved that 1 in 180 patients died in the cottage hospital, as compared to 1 in 30 in the city. He quoted a country doctor as saying, "I would consider it my duty to undertake a formidable operation in a colliery row rather than send a patient to hospital". Simpson himself remarked that "a man laid on an operating table in one of our surgical hospitals is exposed to more chances of death than the English soldier on the field at Waterloo". Three out of five patients died in Paris after surgical treatment at this time.

The subject of hospital improvement was not new. Sir John Pringle, an Edinburgh graduate but a Leyden M.D., suggested in 1752 that barracks, jails and hospitals should be better ventilated, and he used the word "antiseptic". Pringle was present at Culloden where there was a new injury to cope with —a cleft skull as a result of the use of the broadsword. He suggested that hospitals should be sanctuaries on both sides, and put the idea across to George III. Much thought had been given to the building of hospitals since those days but still huge numbers of people died in them.

Simpson's approach was that the hospital unit should be the bed and not the ward, and that the ideal situation would be to have every patient in isolation in a little self-contained pavilion.

Simpson devoted an enormous amount of time and energy to obtaining the records returned by hospitals throughout the country, and gathered these together into two elaborate papers that he published in the early summer of 1869. They proved statistically what he had been saying for years. Patients did not die from an operation, but as a result of their surroundings. He rounded off his first paper with these words:

Must the calling of this dismal death roll still go on unchallenged and unchecked? Shall this pitiless and deliberate sacrifice of human life to conditions which are more or less preventable, be continued or arrested? Do not these terrible figures plead eloquently and clamantly for a revision and reform of our existing hospital system?

Simpson had an answer to all critics of his paper. Hospitals should be built on the "Meccano" principle, of iron, so that every few years they could be pulled to bits and a new site chosen. In the event of an epidemic, a new building could be put up in a matter of days, at a cost infinitesimal compared to that of conventional bricks and cement.

On 29 September the *Daily Review* published an address by Simpson on the subject of the new infirmary, now the leading topic of conversation in Edinburgh. In it he called in question the virtues claimed by Syme and the young Lister of carbolic acid as a cure for all ills and pleaded that, "In the construction of our new Infirmary, the great disinfectants and antiseptics that we should alone depend upon are abundance of space, abundance of light and, above all, abundance of fresh pure and ever-changing air to every patient and every ward in the hospital".

The hospital ward is no longer seen in the U.S.A. Each patient is in a bed in a separate room. "The unit we work with is the bed," explained a nursing superintendent to the author in 1970. "Each is self-sufficient with its own individual supplies. Our hospital is built with the revolutionary theory in mind that it can be easily pulled down and readily re-assembled." How Simpson would have enjoyed the joke! He himself so often said that so called "new ideas were usually as old as the hills".

Simpson had a busy winter with another quick trip to Ireland and three days across the Forth to attend a medical conference at St Andrews. Early in the New Year he become involved as a medical witness in the celebrated divorce case that Sir Charles Mordaunt brought against his wife, who was at present in a lunatic asylum. Sir Charles belonged to the "fast" set, and, much to Queen Victorka's horror, the Prince of Waless's name was mentioned in connection with his circle. Albert had tried so hard to educate the Prince, but the young man had never been allowed to enjoy himself, and freedom had gone to his head. He was subpoenaed in the case and twelve letters of his to Lady Mordaunt were produced and read in court.

On Friday, 11 February 1870, Simpson was summoned to London to give his evidence, and he left by train in the evening, taking with him the three bamboo poles joined with cloth hinges that he laid across the seats to turn his carriage into a sleeper. He also carried a lamp that he clamped into the fabric above the seat. No sooner had his man, Jarvis, returned to Queen Street after organising Simpson in the train, when a telegram arrived, announcing the postponement of the trial until the Wednesday, 16 February. Simpson meanwhile reached London then returned to Edinburgh for a busy day of visits before boarding the train once again on the Tuesday. His evidence was taken the next day on behalf of Lady Mordaunt, whom he considered to be suffering from puerperal insanity. He left London on 17 February, stopping at York for dinner with Lord Houghton on the way home.

He was tired on reaching Edinburgh in the early hours of the morning and admitted that a pain in his chest had compelled him to lie on the floor of the carriage for a while during the night. However, he was immediately back at work, and on the twenty-fourth left Edinburgh again to visit a patient in Forfar. He had to wait for the train on Perth station in a bitter wind. He returned, very tired, complaining of the cold and Jarvis had to help him up the steps and into the house. He sat for some time in a chair in the hall, before agreeing to take to his bed, and have a dose of "Hydrate of Chloral".

For three weeks he lay on his back with the pain in his chest coming and going and breathlessness clawing at his throat. He read books, mostly archaeological, although several were about Spain, where he wanted to go "to get warm in the sun" when he was better. On 18 March he tried to write for the first time and sent a long letter to his son, Magnus Retzius. Visitors were welcome. "Chat away," Simpson would say between gasps for air. "Chat away. It cheers me up and keeps me from sleeping."

In the beginning of April he insisted on moving his bed downstairs to the back drawing room, usually so crammed with female patients. "How old am I" he asked his nephew here one morning. "Fifty-nine? Well, I have done some work. I wish I had been busier." On 6 April he asked his nephew Robert to write a codicil to his will and calmly stated that he would soon die.

The same nephew looked in on 10 April on his way to teach at the Sunday School along the road. "Come back", said Simpson, "and stay all night. I do not think I shall be long here, and I should like you to remain to the end. From extreme pain I have not been able to read or even to think much today, but when I think it is of the words 'Jesus only' and really that is all that is needed, is it not?"

The next few days slid into each other and the family, in Victorian style, gathered together for a death. Robert wrote in his diary for 5 May, "Went to Killin and brought Eve home, but he doesn't know us." Sandy, his older brother, came from Bathgate, and sat on the pillow with Simpson's head on his knee.

"Oh, Sandy, Sandy" were the last words that Simpson spoke. On 6 May Robert's diary reads, "Gradually sinking. After dinner I went up to his room—back drawing room—where Aunt Jessie and Miss Grindlay were watching.

"While Aunt and I were whispering together, we heard a longer drawn sigh than usual. Saw he was going. Aunt rang the bell for the others to come up. I moistened his lips and while the others came in his spirit passed away.

"No struggle—no pain"."

As a Presbyterian minister, Dr Dun, said at the grave, "Such men are rare. We cannot hope to see his like again."

Epilogue

PROMPTED BY THE national and international press, the medical profession in London requested that Simpson's body be interred in Westminster Abbey. They were anxious that the highest possible mark of respect should be paid "to the memory of one whose career had shed such a lustre on the profession". The Dean of Westminster consented and the doctors arranged to defray all the expenses of a public funeral, including the removal of the body from Edinburgh. Lady Simpson, however, declined the offer, saying that she wanted to think of her husband lying beside the children, so the funeral was in Edinburgh.

The Medical Council for the country then held a special meeting, presided over by the Earl of Dalhousie, to decide on a national memorial for Simpson. They then announced that they had agreed on the following: "First, a monument and a statue in Edinburgh; second, a marble bust in Westminster Abbey; third, a hospital in Edinburgh for the diseases of women, constructed on those principles which Sir James so often and so clearly expressed; fourth similar hospitals in London and Dublin should sufficient funds be obtained."

Although the Simpson family had declined the offer for Sir James' burial in Westminster Abbey, they agreed to a memorial. Only fourteen medical men are commemorated there, but of these, six are natives of Scotland. The first was John Woodward born in 1665, professor of physic at Gresham College. He wrote extensively on geology and natural history, and once took part in a duel outside the gates of the Royal College of Physicians in Warwick Lane. The last medical name to be inscribed is that of Joseph Lister.

Walter took his mother, Jessie, away from 52 Queen Street to escape the avalanche of letters of condolence that poured in from America, the Contient, India and of course, England, as well as thousands from all over Scotland. They went to the village of Killin, at the head of Loch Tay, below the slopes of Ben Lawers where the children had often spent holidays in a cottage that belonged to Lady Blantyre. On 17 June Jessie could cope with life no longer, and died at Killin. She was laid in the Warriston grave, alongside her children and hysband.

The words that Simpson had carved in stone for his first child, little Maggie—"Nevertheless—I live"—now stood for so many of the family—four children and both parents. Above the inscription on the obelisk is engraved a butterfly with opening wings.

SELECT BIBLIOGRAPHY

In addition to the books listed below, use was made of the newspapers current in Simpson's day, particularly the *Scotsman*, the *Courant*, *The Times*, the *Edinburgh Review* and *Punch*.

The medical journals of the time were freely consulted, in particular the *Edinburgh Journal of Medical Sciences*, the *Medical Times and Gazette*, the *Lancet*, the *Dublin Medical Journal*, the *Edinburgh Hospital Report*, the *London Medical Gazette*, the *Associated Medical Journal* (later the *British Medical Journal*); and also contemporary issues of the *Journal of Obstetrics and Gynaecology of the British Empire*.

Many more volumes were used for verification of some particular point. The following, however, were the major sources of reference. Simpson's own works are listed separately.

Adams, F., *The Genuine Works of Hippocrates;* The Sydenham Society, London 1849.

Anderson, John, *History of Edinburgh*; Edinburgh 1856.

Anderson, William, *The Poor of Edinburgh and Their Homes*; Edinburgh 1867.

Alison, W. P., *The Management of the Poor in Scotland*; Edinburgh 1840.

Aveling, J. H., *English Midwives, Their History and Prospects*; J. & A. Churchill, London 1872.

Barbour, Margaret F., *Golden Vials;* Edinburgh 1871.

Bell, E., *Storming the Citadel; the story of the woman doctors;* Constable, London 1953.

Bell, George, *Day & Night in the Wynds of Edinburgh*; Edinburgh 1849.

Blackwell, Dr Elizabeth, *Pioneer Work in Opening the Medical Profession to Women*; Longmans, London and New York 1895.

Blake, Dr Sophia Jex, *Medical Women*; Oliphant, Anderson and Ferrier, Edinburgh 1886.

Boston Medical and Surgical Journal, 1846–47 (bound volume).

Bowditch, Nathaniel, *History of the Massachusetts General Hospital*, Boston 1872.

Brown, Dr John, *Horaet Subsecivae*; A. & C. Black, London 1900.

Browne, O'D., *The Rotunda Hospital*; E. & S. Livingstone, Edinburgh 1947.

Channing, Walter, *Etherization in Childbirth*; Boston 1848.

Christison, Sir Robert (edited by his sons), *The Life of Sir Robert Christison*; Blackwood, Edinburgh 1896.

Cockburn, Lord, *Memorials of His Time*; T. N. Fonlis, Edinburgh 1910.

Comrie, John D., *History of Scottish Medicine*; Bailliere, Tindall & Cox, London 1932.

Dilling, W. J., "David Waldie; Prophet of Anaesthetic Properties of Chloroform; *Liverpool Medico-Chirurgical Journal*, 1934, XLII.

Duns, Dr J. *Memoirs of Sir J. Young Simpson*; Edmonston & Douglas, Edinburgh 1873.

Flack, Isaac Harvey, *Lawson Tait*, Heinemann, London 1949.

Flack, Isaac Harvey, *Eternal Eve;* Heinemann, London 1950.

Flagg, J. F. B., *Ether and Chloroform*; Lindsay and Blackiston, Philadelphia 1851.

Findley, P., *Priests of Lucina*; Little, Brown, Boston 1939.

Fyfe, *Scottish Diaries and Memoirs*; Aeneas Mackay, Stirling.

Gordon, Henry Laing, *Sir James Simpson*; Unwin, London 1897.

Grant, Lady Elizabeth of Rothiemurchus, *Memoirs of a Highland Lady*, John Murray, London 1911.

Grant, James, *Old and New Edinburgh;* Cassells, London 1882.

Guthrie, Dr D., *History of Medicine*; Nelson, London 1945.

Haldane, G. S., *Scotland of Our Fathers*; Alexander Maclehose, London 1933.

Harris, Seale, *Woman's Surgeon: Marion Simms*; MacMillan, New York 1950.

Homes, O. W., "The Contagiousness of Puerperal Fever"; *Quarterly Journal of Medicine and Surgery*, 1842.

Hume, Ruth F., *Great Women in Medicine*; Random House, New York 1964.

Long, Crawford Williamson, "An Account of the First Use of Sulphuric Ether"; *Southern Medical and Surgical Journal*, Atlanta 1849 (V. 705, 13).

Longford, Elizabeth, *Victoria, R.I.*, Weidenfeld & Nicolson, London, 1964.

Lutyens, Mary, *Millais and the Ruskins*; John Murray, London 1967.

MacKay, Stewart, *Lawson Tait, His Life and Work*; Bailliere, Tindall and Cox, London 1922.

Manton, Jo., *Elizabeth Garrett Anderson*; Methuen, London 1965.

Marwick, W. H., *Economic Developments in Victorian Scotland*; Pamphlet 1936.

Meigs, Charles, *Obstetrics, The Science and the Art*; Lea & Blanchard, 1849.

Morton, William T. G., *Remarks on the Proper Mode of Administering Sulphuric Ether;* Boston 1847.

Morton, William T. G., collected by C. M. G. Comac; Letters articles, communications and papers; 1909.

Munro, Kerr. Johnstone & Phillips; *Historical Review of British Obstetrics and Gynaecology;* E. & S. Livingstone, Edinburgh 1954.

Paterson, Robert, *Memorials of Professor Syme*; Edmonston & Douglas, Edinburgh 1874.

Power, D'Arcy, *British Masters of Medicine*; Medical Press 1936.

Robinson, Victor M. D., *Victory over Pain*; Schuman, New York 1946.

Ryan, Michael, *Manual of Midwifery*; Renshaw & Rush, London 1931.

Ryder, Corporal, *Four years service in India*; Wm. Burton, Leicester 1853.

Shepherd, John A., *Spencer Wells*; E. & S. Livingstone, Edinburgh 1965.

Simpson, A. R., *Memoirs of Sir James Young Simpson* (Edinburgh Medical Journal) Oliver & Boyd, Edinburgh 1911.

Simpson, E. B., *Sir James Young Simpson*; Oliphant Anderson & Ferrier, London 1896.

Simpson, E. B., *Sir James Young Simpson*; Oliphant Anderson & Ferrier, London 1896.

Simms, Marion, *The Story of My Life*; Appleton, New York, 1885.

Sinclair, W. S., *Semmelweis, his life and work*; University Press, Manchester 1909.

K

Smellie, W., *A Collection of Preternatural cases and observations in Midwifery*; D. Wilson and T. Durham, London 1764.

Smith, Truman, *An Examination of the Question of Anaesthesia*; New York 1859.

Snow, John, *On the inhalation of the Vapour of Ether*; London, 1847.

Snow, John, *On Chloroform and other Anaesthetics*; London 1858.

Stokes, William, *The life of George Petrie*; Longmans, London 1868.

Sykes, W. S., *Essays on the 1st 100 years of Anaesthesia*; E. & S. Livingstone, Edinburgh 1960.

Thoms, Herbert, *Classical Contributions to Obstetrics and Gynaecology*; Chas. C. Thomas, Illinois 1935.

Todd, Margaret, *The Life of Sophia Jex Blake*; Macmillan, London 1918.

Turner, L., *The Story of a Great Hospital, Royal Infirmary, Edinburgh*; Oliver and Boyd, Edinburgh 1937.

Wise, R. Staunton, *12 months experience of the benefits of chloroform in Midwifery*; Longman, London 1849.

Wilson, T. G., *Victorian Doctor*; Fischer, New York 1946.

Wyatt, Henry, *William Harvey*; Leonard Parsons, London 1924.

*   *   *

THE PUBLISHED WORKS OF JAMES YOUNG SIMPSON

It is not claimed that this list is comprehensive. The works are drawn up in chronological order.

"Pathological observations on the diseases of the placenta". Part I: "Congestion and inflammation". Edinburgh, J. Stark, 1835.
Repr. from *Edinb. M. & S. J.*, 1836, xlv.

"On the evidence of the occasional contagious propagation of malignant cholera, which is derived from cases of its direct importation into new localities by infected individuals". Edinburgh, J. Stark, 1838.
Repr. from *Edinb. M. & S. J.*, 1838, xlix.

"Contributions to intra-uterine pathology". Part I: "Notices of cases of peritonitis in the foetus in utero". Edinburgh, J. Stark, 1838.
Repr. from *Edinb. M. & S. J.*, 1838, 1.

The same. Part II. "On the inflammatory origin of some varieties of hernia and malformation in the foetus". Edinburgh, J. Stark, 1839.
Repr. from: *Edinb. M. & S. J.*, 1839, lii.

Short syllabus of the course of lectures on obstetric medicine. Edinburgh, T. Allan & Co., 1839.

"[Letter] to the honourable Sir James Forrest, of Comiston, Bart., Lord Provost of the city of Edinburgh". Edinburgh 1840.

"List of the preparations, casts, drawings, instruments, obstetric machinery, etc., contained in [his] museum and employed by him in the illustration of his lectures on midwifery". Edinburgh, T. Allan & Co., 1840.

"Case of amputation of the neck of the womb, folllwed by pregnancy; with remarks on the pathology and radical treatment of the cauliflower excrescence from the os uteri". Edinburgh, J. Stark, 1841.
Repr. from *Edinb. M. & S. J.*, 1841, xiv.

"Memorial on the propriety of continuing the chair of general pathology; submitted to the right hon. the Lord Provost, magistrates, and members of the town council, composing the college committee of the patrons of the University of Edinburgh". Edinburgh, T. Allan & Co., 1841.

"Postscript to Dr Simpson's memorial on the propriety of continuing the chair of general pathology". Edinburgh 1841.

"Antiquarian notices of leprosy and leper hospitals in Scotland and England". Part I. Edinburgh, J. Stark, 1841.
Repr. from *Edinb. M. & S. J.*, 1841, lvi.

The same. Part II: "The nosological nature of the disease". Edinburgh, J. Stark, 1842.
Repr. from *Edinb. M. & S. J.*, 1842, lvii.

The same. Part III: "The etiological history of the disease". Edinburgh, J. Stark 1842.
Repr. from *Edinb. M. & S. J.*, 1842, lvii.

"Remarks on the conduct and duties of young physicians;

addressed to the Edinburgh medical graduates of 1842".
Edinburgh, Maclachlan, Stewart & Co., 1842.

The same, 2nd ed. Edinburgh, Maclachlan, Stewart & Co.,
1848.

"Contributions to the pathology and treatment of diseases of
the uterus". Part I: "Propositions regarding uterine diagnosis". Edinburgh, Balfour & Jack, 1843.
Repr. from *Month, J. M. Sc.*, Lond. & Edinb., 1843, iii.

The same. Part III: "On the measurement of the cavity of the
uterus as a means of diagnosis in some of the morbid states of
that organ". Edinburgh, 1843.
Repr. from *Month. J. M. Sc.*, Lond. & Edinb., 1843, iii.

"On the alleged infecundity of females born co-twins with
males; with notes on the average proportion of marriages
without issue in general society". Edinburgh, Stark & Co.,
1844.
Repr. from *Edinb. M. & S. J.*, 1844, lxi.

"Memoir on the sex of the child as a cause of difficulty and
danger in human parturition". Edinburgh, Stark & Co.,
1844.
Repr. from *Edinb. M. & S. J.*, 1844, lxii.

"On the expulsion and extraction of the placenta before the
child in placental presentations'. (Worcester, Deighton &
Co., 1845).
Repr. from *Prov. M. & S. J.*, Lond., 1845.

"On the Detachment and extraction of the placenta in cases of
unavoidable haemorrhage". Reply to Dr Radford. (Worcester, Deighton & Co., 1845.
Repr. from *Prov. M. & S. J.*, Lond., 1845.

"Some remarks on the treatment of unavoidable haemorrhage
by extraction of the placenta before the child. With a few
observations on Dr Lee's objections to the practice". (With
correspondence with Dr Ramsbotham.) London, 1845.
Repr. from *Lond. M. Gaz.*, 1845, n.s., i.

"Additional observations on unavoidable haemorrhage in cases
of placental presentation". London, Wilson & Ogilvy, 1845.
Repr. from *Lond. M. Gaz.*, 1845, n.s., i.

"Clinical lectures on midwifery and the diseases of women and
children". Taken in shorthand by Charles D. Arnott.
London, 1845.

ANCHOR

Repr. from *Month. J. M. Sc.*, Lond. & Edinb., 1845, v.

"Clinical lectures on midwifery and the diseases of women and infants during the session 1845–6". Edinburgh, H. Paton, 1846.

Repr. from *North. J. M.*, Edinb., 1846, iv.

"Observations regarding, the influence of galvanism upon the action of the uterus during labour". Edinburgh, Sutherland & Knox, 1846.

Repr. from *Month. J. M. Sc.*, Lond. & Edinb., 1846, vi.

"Ovariotomy; is it or is it not an operation justifiable upon the common principles of surgery? Are or are not capital operations in surgery justifiable to the extent generally practised?" Edinburgh, Sutherland & Knox, 1846.

Repr. from *Month. J. M. Sc.*, Lond. & Edinb., 1846, vi.

"Some suggestions regarding the anatomical source and pathological nature of post-partum haemorrhage". Edinburgh, H. Paton, 1846.

Repr. from *North J. M.* Edinb., 1846, vi.

"Anaesthetic and other therapeutic properties of chloroform". Edinburgh, Sutherland & Knox, 1847.

Repr. from *Month. J. M. Sc.*, Lond. & Edinb., 1847–8, viii.

"Answer to the religious objections advanced against the employment of anaesthetic agents in midwifery and surgery". Edinburgh, Sutherland & Knox, 1847.

"Notes on the inhalation of sulphuric ether in the practice of midwifery". Edinburgh, Sutherland & Knox, 1847.

Repr. from *Month J. M. Sc.*, Lond. & Edinb., 1846–7, n.s., i.

"Remarks on the superinduction of anaesthesia in natural and morbid parturition; with cases illustrative of the use and effects of chloroform in obstetric practice". Edinburgh, Sutherland & Knox, 1847.

The same. With an appendix. Boston, W. B. Little & Co., 1848.

Notice of a new anaesthetic agent as a substitute for sulphuric ether in surgery and midwifery; commnuicated to the Medico-Chirurgical Society of Edinburgh at their meeting on 10th November 1847". Edinburgh, Sutherland & Knox, 1847.

The same, reprinted Edinburgh, Sutherland & Knox, 1847.

The same, reprinted, 4,000 copies. Edinburgh, Sutherland & Knox, 1848.

The same. New York, Rushton, Clark & Co., 1848.

The same, reprinted twice. New York, Rushton, Clark & Co., 1848.

"On solutions of gun cotton, gutta percha, and caoutchouc as dressing for wounds, etc." London, 1848.
Repr. from *London. M. Gaz.* 1848, n.s., vii.

"Anaesthetic midwifery; report on its early history and progress". Edinburgh, Sutherland & Knox, 1848.
Repr. from *Month. J. M. Sc.*, Edinb. 1848, ix.

The same. Edinburgh, Sutherland & Knox, 1848.
Repr. from *Prov. M. & S. J.*, Lond., 1848, xii.

"Letter in reply to Dr Collins, on the duration of labour as a cause of danger and mortality to the mother and infant". Worcester, Deighton & Co., 1848.
Repr. from *Prov. M. & S. J.*, Lond., 1848, xii.

"Local anaesthesia; notes on its artificial production by chloroform, etc., in the lower animals and in man". Worcester, Deighton & Co., 1848.
Repr. from *Prov. M. & S. J.*, Lond., 1848, xii.

"Obstetrical statistics, etc." A second letter in reply to Dr Collins. Edinburgh, Sutherland & Knox, 1848.

"On the diagnosis and treatment of retroversion of the unimpregnated uterus". Dublin, Hodges & Smith, 1848.
Repr. from *Q.J.M.Sc.*, Dublin, 1848, v.

"Remarks on the alleged fatal case of chloroform inhalation". Edinburgh, Murray & Gibb, 1848.
Repr. from *Lancet*, Lond., 1848, i.

"Report of the Einburgh Royal Maternity Hospital from 1844 to 1846. (Being an analysis of the obstetric practice of the institution for the first two years)". Edinburgh, Sutherland & Knox, 1848.
Repr. from *Month. J. M. Sc.*, Lond. & Edinb. 1848–9, ix.

"Some remarks on the value and necessity of the numerical or statistical method of inquiry as applied to various questions in operative surgery". Edinburgh, Sutherland & Knox, 1848.
Repr. from *Month. J. M. Sc.*, Lond. & Edinb., 1847–9, viii.

"Anaesthesia; or, the employment of chloroform and ether in surgery, midwifery, etc. Philadelphia, Lindsay & Blakiston, 1849.

"The attitude and positions, natural and preternatural, of the

foetus in utero, acts of the reflex or excito-motory system".
Edinburgh, Sutherland & Knox, 1849.

Repr. from *Month. J. M. Sc.*, Lond. & Edinb., 1848–9, ix.

The same. Parts I & II. Edinburgh, Sutherland & Knox, 1849.

"On a suction-tractor, or new mechanical power, as a substitute
for the forceps in tedious labours". Edinburgh, Sutherland
& Knox, 1849.

Repr. from *Edinb. Month. J. M. Sc.*, 1848–9, ix.

"Two notices of the obstetric air tractor". Edinburgh, Sutherland & Knox, 1849.

Repr. from *Edinb. Month. J. M. Sc.*, 1848–9 ix.

"Memoir on turning, as an alternative for craniotomy and the
long forceps, in deformity of the brim of the pelvis, etc."
Worcester, Deighton & Co., 1850.

"On the detection and treatment of intra-uterine polypi".
Edinburgh, Sutherland & Knox, 1850.

Repr. from *Edinb. Month. J. M. Sc.*,, 1850, x.

"Speech at the medico-Chirurgical Society relative to homoeopathy; with notes on the peculiar theological opinions of
some disciples of Hahnemann, etc." Edinburgh, Sutherland
& Knox, 1851.

The same. "Homoeopathy. Speech at the medico-chirurgical
Society, etc." 2nd ed. Edinburgh, Sutherland & Knox,
1852.

The same. "Homoeopathy; its tenets and tendencies, theoretical,
theological, and therapeutical". Edinburgh, Sutherland &
Knox, 1853.

The same. 1. Am. from 3. Edinb. ed. Philadelphia, Lindsay &
Blakiston, 1854.

"Contributions to obstetric pathology and practice". Edinburgh, Sutherland & Knox, 1853.

"The modern advancement of practical medicine and surgery;
an inaugural address to the Medico-Chirurgical Society of
Edinburgh". Edinburgh (Murray & Gibbs, 1853).

Repr. from *Month. J. M. Sc.*, Lond. & Edinb. 1853, xvi.

"On anaesthetics in instrumental and natural parturition; in
a letter to Prof. Meigs, of Philadelphia". London, I. Richards,
1853.

"Pathological observations on puerperal, arterial obstruction
and inflammation". Edinburgh, 1854.

"Regarding the History and effects of Chloroform." *Encyclopaedia Brittanica* vol. ii, 1855.

The obstetric memoirs and contributions of J. Y. Simpson. Ed. by W. O. Priestley and Horatio R. Storer, 2. v. Philadelphia, J. B., Lippincott & Co., 1855–6.

"Notes on some ancient Greek medical vases for containing lykion; and on the modern use of the same drug in India". Edinburgh, Sutherland & Knox, 1856.

"Physicians and Physic; three addresses. I. On the duties of young physicians. II. On the prospects of young physicians. III. On the modern advancement of physic". Edinburgh, A. & C. Black, 1856.

"Was the Roman army provided with medical officers?" Edinburgh, Sutherland & Knox, 1856.

The same. "Des médicins attachés aux armées romaines. Trad. de l'anglais et augmenté d'une note additionnelle par C.–A. Buttura". Paris, E. Thunot, 1857.
    Repr. from: *Gaz. med. de Par.*, 1857, xxviii.

"Acupressure; a new method of arresting surgical haemorrhage". Edinburgh, 1860.
    Repr. from: *Edinb. M.J.* 1859–60, v.

The same. Edinburgh, 1860.

"On acupressure in amputations; with illustrative cases". London, 1860.
    Repr. from *Med. Times & Gaz.*, Lond., 1860, i.

"Cases of amputations with acupressure". London, 1860.
    Repr. from *Med. Times & Gaz.*, Lond., 1860, i.

"Archaeology; its past and its future work. Being the annual address to the Society of Antiquaries of Scotland". Edinburgh, Edmonston & Douglas, 1861.

Clinical lectures on diseases of women. Philadelphia, Blanchard & Lea, 1863.

"On the anatomical type of structure of the human umbilical cord and placenta". Edinburgh, Neill & Co., 1863.
    Repr. from *Tr. Roy. Soc.* Edinb., 1863, xxiii, pt. ii.

The same. Edinburgh, R. Clark, 1864.

"Acupressure; a new method of arresting surgical haemorrhage and of accelerating the healing of wounds". Edinburgh, A. & C. Black, 1864.

"Answers to the various objections against acupressure or the temporary metallic compression of arteries, adduced by Professors Miller, Erichsen, Nendorfer, Spence, Feruon, and Syme". Edinburgh, 1864.

Repr. from his: Acupressure. Edinb., 1864.

"Comparison of the ligature and acupressure as haemostatic agents; tabulated contrast between them". Edinburgh, 1864.

Repr. from his: Acupressure. Edinb. 1864.

Conversazione of the Lothians' Medical Association; address by J. Y. Simpson. Edinburgh, Oliver & Boyd, 1867.

Repr. from *Edinb. M.J.*, 1866–7, xii.

"Note on the history of carbolic acid and its compounds in surgery prior to 1867". London, 1867.

Repr. from *Lancet*, London., 1867, ii.

"Notes on the progress of acupressure". Edinburgh, A. & C. Black, 1867.

The same. 2nd ed. Edinburgh, A. & C. Black, 1867.

Medical graduation address, 1 August 1868. Edinburgh, 1868.

The same. "Address to the Edinburgh medical graduates, August 1, 1868". Edinburgh, Oliver & Boyd, 1868.

Repr. from *Edinb. M.J.*, 1868–9, xiv.

"Proposal to stamp out small-pox and other contagious disease". Edinburgh, Edmonston & Douglas, 1868.

Repr. from *Med. Times & Gaz.*, Lond., 1868, i.

The same. 2nd ed. Edinburgh, Edmonston & Douglas, 1868.

Repr. from *Med. Times & Gaz.*, London, 1868, i.

"Hospitalism; its effects on the results of surgical operations, etc." Edinburgh, Oliver & Boyd, 1869.

Repr. from *Edinb. M.J.*, 1869–70, xv.

Part I: "Country amputation statistics". Part II: "2098 country amputations; 2089 hospital amputations". Part III: "3077 provincial hospital amputations".

"On the relative danger to life from limb amputations in St. Bartholomew's Hospital, London, and country practice". London, 1869.

Repr. from *Brit. M.J.*, Lond., 1869, i.

"Historical letter on the introduction of anaesthetics in dentistry and surgery in America and on their first employment in midwifery in Great Britain". London, 1870.

Repr. from *Med. Times & Gaz.*, Lond., 1870, i.

"History of modern anaesthetics". A second letter to Dr Jacob
   Bigelow. Edinburgh, Edmondston & Douglas, 1870.
"Therapeutic note on chloral". London, 1870.
   Repr. from *Med. Times & Gaz.*, Lond., 1870, i.
A reply to Dr Jacob Bigelow's second letter. (Anaesthetics.)
   19 pp. Boston, 1870.
   Suppl. to: *J. Gynaec. Soc.*, Bost., 1870, ii.
Works of J. Y. Simpson, 3 vols., Edinburgh, A. & C. Black,
   1871–2.

Simpson's Archaeological Works:

"The Cat Stane (Edinburghshire)". 1862.
"Antiquarian Notices of Syphilis in Scotland". 1862.
"Notes on Scottish Magical Charm Stones". 1863.
"Ancient Cave Sculpturings in Fife". 1864.
The above were later collected into three volumes, published in
   Edinburgh in 1872.

Other works include:

"Is the great Pyramid of Gezah a Meterological Mound?"
"Sir D. Brewster—his last days and death".
"Dead in Trespasses and Sins".
Hymn "Stop and Think".
Poems—private publications 1852 and 1868.

Index